TRANSFORMING PRESIDENTIAL HEALTHCARE

Ensuring Comprehensive Care for the Commander in Chief amid 21st Century Threats

JEFFREY KUHLMAN, MD, MPH

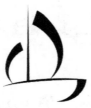

Ballast Books, LLC
www.ballastbooks.com

Copyright © 2024 by Jeffrey Kuhlman

The views expressed in this publication are those of the author and do not necessarily reflect the
official policy or position of the Department of Defense or the US government. The public release
clearance of this publication by the Department of Defense does not imply Department of Defense
endorsement or factual accuracy of the material.

ISBN: 978-1-964934-15-0

Printed in the United States of America

Published by Ballast Books
www.ballastbooks.com

For more information, bulk orders, appearances, or speaking requests,
please email: info@ballastbooks.com

To my parents, Henry and Patricia Kuhlman;
to my children: Michael, Isabella, Lena, and Henry;
and to my wife, Sandy Montaperto Kuhlman—
you are the purpose of life and give my life purpose.

CONTENTS

THE HONOR OF A LIFETIME

Think back to March 30, 1981. Do you remember where you were that day? I do.

I grew up outside of Chattanooga in Collegedale, Tennessee. One day at about 2:30 p.m., I was on my way to Little Debbie, where I drove a forklift for a few years to put myself through high school and college. I heard on the car radio that shots had been fired at President Ronald Reagan.

Later, we found out that the president had been walking out of the Washington Hilton when an assailant fired six shots at him. A Secret Service agent threw his body in harm's way and Mr. Reagan's protective detail hustled him into the presidential limo, "The Beast." Jerry Parr, the Secret Service Special Agent in Charge (SAIC), jumped on top of him and asked, "Hey, did you get hit?"

"No, I'm fine, I'm fine," the president replied.

Whenever shots were fired in the vicinity of the president, the standing Secret Service plan was to rush back to Crown, the code name for the White House. At the time, the White House physician, if part of the in-town movements, had no pre-hospital trauma training or equipment. Apparently, everyone thought, *What could ever happen to the president in D.C.?*

That day, the Beast flew down Connecticut Avenue. As the car sped under the Dupont Circle overpass, Jerry Parr saw a drop of blood on the corner of President Reagan's mouth and declared, "Forget this. We're going to GW [the George Washington University Hospital]." Dr. Daniel Ruge, the physician to the president at the time, was not part of the evacuation and had to jump in a trailing official vehicle. He caught up to the president only after Mr. Reagan had been assessed and stabilized by emergency staff.

GW is on Twenty-Third Street instead of Sixteenth (as in 1600 Pennsylvania Avenue). When the Beast rolled up to GW, President Reagan walked in under his own power. No one except those inside saw that he groaned and his knees buckled. The emergency medical nurses and three surgical resident physicians, with recent trauma training at Shock Trauma in Baltimore, saved his life that day because they treated him like any other patient. They laid him down, a nurse jumped up on top and cut off his clothes, and they prepared him for resuscitation, further evaluation, and surgery.

It soon became clear that a .22-caliber bullet had ricocheted off the limo's bulletproof exterior, striking the president under his left arm, puncturing a lung, and causing significant internal bleeding. In fact, during his stay at the hospital, the president lost about 3.7 quarts of blood. The shooter, John Hinckley Jr., was trying to impress actress Jodie Foster. He also managed to severely wound White House press secretary James Brady in the head, along with a Washington police officer named Thomas Delahanty and Secret Service agent Tim McCarthy, who wasn't even supposed to be working that day. McCarthy had drawn the short straw and had to fill in for someone else. He had spread his body over the president's and taken a bullet in the chest, which probably saved Reagan's life. Both McCarthy and Delahanty recovered fully, but Brady remained disabled for the rest of his life until his death in 2014.

President Reagan's injuries turned out to be much worse than initially thought. In fact, the bullet came within millimeters of his pulmonary vasculature—a bit more than an inch from his heart and an inch from his aorta—something that became apparent only moments before doctors rushed him into surgery. That's when Mr. Reagan famously quipped to his doctors, "Hey, I hope you guys are Republicans."

But this was D.C., where very few Republicans make their home.

Fortunately for the president, the GW doctors were emergency medicine nurses and physicians experienced in emergency room trauma. Mr. Reagan lived because they treated him like a trauma patient, not like a VIP. Just before they wheeled him into the operating room, they replied, "Oh, Mr. President, today we are all Republicans."

And then the surgeons and OR nurses and techs worked together to save the president's life.

The CEO of the George Washington University Hospital happened to be out of the country that day, and the White House press secretary was incapacitated. So who would stand up in a press conference to let the nation know what had happened? That duty quickly fell to Dennis S. O'Leary, a hematologist and the chief of clinical affairs at GW. According to a *Washington Post* article, "As the presidential motorcade was roaring toward the hospital, someone mentioned to O'Leary that 'the president' was on the way. 'The president of what?' he said, unaware of the shooting."[1] For two weeks, O'Leary kept the world informed about the president's brush with death.

At the time, I was within a couple of weeks of graduating from high school. I clearly remember Dr. O'Leary getting up and, in his distinct baritone voice, making clear, no-nonsense, factual statements about GW's famous presidential patient. He later became the CEO of the Joint Commission, a non-profit organization that accredits and certifies healthcare organizations and programs in the US and internationally. He died in early 2023.

The Reagan assassination attempt altered the entire trajectory of the White House Medical Unit. Much of this book is about those changes. But back in 1981, as I heard about the incident on the radio, my teenage brain thought, *Oh, that's pretty cool. There are doctors and nurses who care for the president.*

Little did I know that one day I would serve among them.

EVERY DAY A HISTORIC DAY

Every day spent caring for the president, whether in D.C. or abroad, is a historic day. Exciting things happen. Some days are more historic and challenging than others, of course. Events such as 9/11 and the subsequent elimination of Osama bin Laden a decade later tend to overshadow most other occasions. But overseeing the physical, mental, and even spiritual well-being of the president of the United States, as well as caring for many others who work closely with him, creates an unforgettable experience.

I was privileged to have a front-row seat to watch significant world events unfold during the terms of three US presidents: Bill Clinton, George W. Bush, and Barack Obama. During that crucial period, the office and duties of the physician to the president underwent important and noteworthy changes. For Presidents Clinton and Bush, I served on the White House Medical Unit staff in various capacities, while President Obama chose me to serve as the physician to the president during his first term in office (2009–2013).

I did not write *Transforming Presidential Healthcare* as a personal memoir so much as an insider's history of the crucial ways in which medical care has advanced in the recent past for the president, his immediate family, and those who work with him in various capacities throughout the eighteen-acre complex on which the White House sits. As you might expect, the medical care of the US president has come a long way since a newly inaugurated George Washington became ill and someone suggested that it might be a good idea to have a physician available. Dr. James Craik, a former regimental surgeon in the Continental Army whom Washington had met as a lieutenant colonel, soon got the job. He visited Washington in New York and

Mount Vernon whenever summoned, right up until Washington's death on December 14, 1799.

As we'll see, some of the most significant changes protecting the president were put in place after the attempt on President Reagan's life. After the turn of the century, changes to presidential medicine have accelerated. Physicians connected to the White House have expanded their care far beyond annual physicals to encompass anything from protective medicine to care of cabinet members, whole person care, dealing with asymmetrical threats, special situations, crises, and more.

What does it take to become the physician to the president? While I suppose some individuals dream of taking on such a role early in their lives, I confess that I didn't. I never had any plans to become the physician to the president and not once did I set my sights on securing the position. I joined the navy out of a desire to serve my country and to pay for my medical education. The rest just unfolded over time.

How grateful I am, however, for those amazing years I spent working around, in, and for the White House! From 2000 to 2013, I served as a member of the White House Medical Unit, worked as the director of the White House Medical Unit, and finally spent four and a half years as the physician to the president. In that time, I took hundreds of trips around the world in support of the presidents, traveled to more than ninety countries, and helped upgrade the medical care provided for those working on the Eighteen Acres. I had the privilege of working with first-class medical professionals and serving the men and women who help keep this country and world moving in a positive direction.

In *Transforming Presidential Healthcare*, I tell some memorable stories, describe the critical work of the White House Medical Unit, explain how and why we must constantly upgrade the medical care we provide to keep up with a host of contemporary challenges, and discuss the physical and mental requirements essential for any US president in the twenty-first century.

I want to be clear that this is *not* a tell-all book, nor is it filled with salacious stories about illicit or questionable activities taking place behind closed doors. If you're looking for that kind of material, I recommend that you search elsewhere. I promised each of the presidents I served that I would never betray their healthcare or their personal privacy. That promise still holds today, a decade after I left my post at the White House. I also assured each of the presidents I served that I would adhere strictly to my personal mantra: No politics, no policy, just trusted medical advice.

To Presidents Clinton, Bush, and Obama, I say thank you for trusting me with such an important role in your healthcare during your time in office. To the many others who lived or worked on the Eighteen Acres, I say thank you for helping to make my job so rewarding, enjoyable, and, yes, at times challenging and exciting. It was the great honor of my life to serve alongside all of you.

JEFFREY KUHLMAN, MD, MPH
Captain, Flight Surgeon,
Medical Corps, US Navy (Retired)
Orlando, Florida
January 30, 2024

PART ONE

——◆——

THE PRESIDENTS

1

WHY DO PRESIDENTS NEED THEIR OWN DOCTORS?

All US presidents since George Washington have had a personal physician attending to their medical needs. Until the twentieth century, however, those physicians were both part-time and unofficial. Not until 1901 did the position become full-time, and not until 1928 did the title "physician to the president" become official through an act of Congress. The core responsibility of the physician to the president is to provide and/or oversee primary care for the chief executive and his family, and to integrate any necessary pre-hospital care with the Secret Service.

Some people may wonder why a president needs his or her own doctor in the first place. They may think, *I don't have my own personal physician. Why shouldn't the president get healthcare in the same way I do?*

It's a good question, and a fair one. Not only is the president an important figure for national and international geopolitical stability, but he also faces greater potential threats to his health beyond the everyday challenges of illness.

A Crucial Leader

Since the end of the nineteenth century at least, the president of the United States has occupied a key leadership role alongside the leaders of other key world powers. After the twentieth century's two world wars, that leadership role only grew.

Today, the president of the United States leads the third most populous nation in the world after China and India. The president is the acknowledged leader of the free world's 1.6 billion citizens, is the commander in chief of the most potent military force on the globe, and shepherds the largest economy in the world with a gross domestic product of $25.4 trillion (compared to China's $17.9 trillion and Japan's $4.2 trillion).

For all these reasons and many others like them, it is imperative to expend great effort to keep the US president as safe and in as good health as possible. Anything less could quickly lead to chaos not only in this nation of more than 333 million citizens but also throughout the world and its current 8 billion inhabitants. In the modern era, the role of the physician to the president, and that of the medical staff serving the White House, is simply indispensable.

A Brief History of White House Medicine

When George Washington took office as US president in 1789, he relied on his personal physician, comrade-in-arms, and close friend, Army Colonel James Kraik, to serve as the physician general (precursor to the surgeon general) and as the physician to the president. For the next century, whenever a president needed medical care, senior military physicians (the surgeon general of either the army or the navy) were most often called upon.

President Grover Cleveland appointed George Sternberg as surgeon general of the army in 1893 and promoted him to the rank of brigadier general. During his nine-year tenure, Dr. Sternberg, a prominent bacteriologist, would occasionally provide medical care to the president. He mentored Dr. Walter Reed (after whom the Walter Reed

General Hospital was named in 1909) and was influential in the suppression of typhoid and yellow fever.

US Navy Captain Presley Rixey was appointed physician to the Executive Mansion in 1898 to provide medical care for President William McKinley. Epileptic seizures in 1873 had rendered Mrs. McKinley an invalid, requiring almost continuous medical care. President McKinley preferred the services of a personal physician whose primary responsibilities focused on the president and the First Lady without the demands placed on a surgeon general.

When President McKinley was fatally shot in 1901, Captain Rixey was not nearby, as he had escorted Mrs. McKinley to the First Family's home in Canton, Ohio. Dr. Rixey hurried to Buffalo, where he directed the president's post-operative care after several surgeons had attempted unsuccessfully to remove the bullet.

The Executive Mansion, once commonly called "the President's House," became known as the White House after President Teddy Roosevelt issued a presidential order in 1901. The first decade of the twentieth century became a time of workspace transition as the West Wing of the White House was built and the first physician was permanently assigned there. Before then, doctors came from their assigned hospitals or offices and examined the president and First Family in their private living quarters, located on the second floor of the White House.

President Roosevelt also permanently assigned Dr. Rixey—who simultaneously served as the surgeon general of the navy, achieving the terminal rank of vice admiral—as the White House physician. Dr. Rixey thus became the first doctor to serve full-time as the White House physician.

The office of attending physician to Congress was established by a congressional resolution in 1928. That same year, Congress also authorized the promotion to colonel of all army doctors assigned as White House physicians. Major James Coupal was the first to be promoted under the statute. Two years later, Congress stipulated that those who served as the physician to the White House should have the temporary rank of colonel (army) or captain (navy), retroactive to March 6, 1929, when Commander Joel T. Boone was assigned to the post by President Hoover. A 1956 act of Congress eliminated the word "temporary" from the designation of rank.

The White House Medical Unit (WHMU) was established in the West Wing in 1945.[2] At times, a doctor's office and exam room (including x-ray shielding) was also in the West Wing, staffed by the WHMU. It relocated to the Old Executive Office Building (OEOB) during the Nixon administration, where it remains today, functioning as a worksite and travel medicine clinic for those working on the Eighteen Acres.

In 1961, President John F. Kennedy appointed the first civilian physician, Janet Travell, to serve as the physician to the president. However, the military continued to have a medical presence, with Navy Captain George Burkley (later vice admiral) serving as physician to the White House until he became the physician to the president when Lyndon B. Johnson took office. Dr. Travell had an office on the ground floor of the White House, while Captain Burkley had his office in the West Wing. From 1961 to 2013, seven of the eleven individuals holding this office were military officers who remained on active duty during their tenure (see Appendix 1 for a full list of physicians to the president since 1901).

HEALTH PROBLEMS OF US PRESIDENTS

As I look through the long lens of history, I think of the first two deaths of a sitting US president. William Henry Harrison died on April 4, 1841, of complications from pneumonia,[3] while Zachary Taylor died on July 9, 1850, allegedly after consuming prodigious amounts of cherries and iced milk.[4] If these men had come into office a hundred years later, both would have had a good chance of surviving. Unfortunately, the contemporary medical interventions of antibiotics, fluid resuscitation, and expanded medical knowledge had not come on the scene in their time.

President Harrison died just thirty-one days after his inauguration at age sixty-eight, while President Taylor died sixteen months into his term at age sixty-five. The death of President Harrison triggered a mini-crisis, as the US Constitution did not make clear whether the vice president would become president upon the death of the sitting president or rather simply become acting president. Vice President John Tyler took the oath of office on April 6, 1841, and Congress passed a joint resolution on May 31 confirming Tyler as president for the remainder of President Harrison's term. That precedent was followed seven times afterward until the passage of Section 1 of the Twenty-Fifth Amendment to the Constitution in 1967 (see chapter 11).

Other presidential deaths followed. Warren G. Harding, the twenty-ninth president, took office in 1921 at the age of fifty-five and died of a heart attack on August 2, 1923, at the age of fifty-seven. Professional disagreements between his personal doctor, Dr. Charles Sawyer, and another White House doctor, Dr. Joel T. Boone, made a tragic situation even worse. Dr. Boone diagnosed underlying heart problems and cited an expert Stanford cardiologist for support. The prevailing wisdom today is that the president had suffered undiagnosed heart attacks and died of congestive heart failure.

Franklin Delano Roosevelt, the only president to serve for more than two terms (he served twelve years, from ages fifty-one to sixty-three), suffered from polio, paralysis, and related complications. In April 1945, he traveled to Warm Springs, Georgia—a frequent rest location for him—and died on April 12 of a cerebral hemorrhage, likely a result of uncontrolled hypertension. History records that Admiral Ross McIntire, an ENT surgeon and the president's physician, failed to recognize hypertension and congestive heart failure until FDR's daughter Anna, who served as his advisor and aide, insisted her father be evaluated at Bethesda Naval Hospital, where Lieutenant Commander Harvey Bruenn, a young, well-trained cardiologist, diagnosed and recommended treatment in the spring of 1944.[5]

Setting aside the extreme cases of deaths in office, presidents have health problems, some of them serious, just like everyone else. Presidents are human, so they come down with the usual maladies common to us all: a sore throat; a cold; an upset stomach; the flu. An experienced primary care physician must identify the real problem and then sort out the right thing to do without overdoing anything.

Consider just a few of the health challenges and scares faced by former US presidents: [6]

- Andrew Jackson (1767–1845) was known for a fierce temper that landed him in multiple duels and fights. One gunfight in 1812 left a lead bullet in his arm that, twenty years later, started giving him severe pain. His surgeon cut open his arm and squeezed out the bullet (all without anesthesia). Not only did the former pain go away, but his general health improved. Could the president have suffered from lead poisoning?

- Grover Cleveland (1837–1908) had doctors remove a cancerous growth from his mouth while on board a friend's yacht. The whole operation was done clandestinely in May 1893 without notifying the press. The president lived another fifteen years and died at age seventy-one of a heart attack.

- William Howard Taft (1857–1930) suffered from obesity; at the end of his presidential term, he weighed about 350 pounds. One popular but apparently apocryphal story says that his enormous girth once got him stuck in a White House bathtub, requiring his doctor to grease him up with butter to extricate him.[7] He suffered from sleep apnea and died in 1930 from a host of related conditions, including heart disease, high blood pressure, and bladder inflammation.

- John Fitzgerald Kennedy (1917–1963) had a sickly childhood, suffering from scarlet fever, diphtheria, and asthma, among other maladies. He also had Addison's disease, a potentially fatal immune system dysfunction. His physician diagnosed the latter illness when Kennedy was about thirty years old and told him he had less than a year to live. Steroids helped JFK manage the disease until his assassination on November 22, 1963.

- Ronald Wilson Reagan (1911–2004) underwent successful procedures for both colon cancer and skin cancer during his second term as president. Doctors diagnosed him with Alzheimer's disease in 1994, five years after he left office. He died ten years later from Alzheimer's and pneumonia.

ASSASSINATION ATTEMPTS

The job of the president of the United States has proven to be a dangerous occupational choice. The world may never know how many times someone, somewhere on the planet, has plotted or attempted to kill a US president.

History records unsuccessful attempts on the lives of Presidents Andrew Jackson, Theodore Roosevelt, Franklin Delano Roosevelt, John F. Kennedy (before his assassination in Dallas, Texas), Richard Nixon, Gerald Ford, Jimmy Carter, Ronald Reagan, George H. W. Bush, Bill Clinton, George W. Bush, Barack Obama, Donald Trump, and Joe Biden. The physician to the president stays within two minutes of the president at all times so that if an attack on the president occurs—incidents that we hope never take place, such as a knife stabbing, gunshot wounds, a heart attack, or falling down stairs and cracking open a head—a medical doctor very familiar with the patient can provide immediate, expert care. The physician to the president works to keep the blood in the body and then executes an existing plan to quickly get the ailing or injured president to definitive care.

Tragically, too many assassination attempts have succeeded. The third president to die in office was the first to die by assassination. President Abraham Lincoln, the nation's sixteenth president, died early in his second term on April 15, 1865, the day after he was shot. Ironically, he had signed legislation just hours before the shooting that established what would become the United States Secret Service, officers dedicated to protecting the president. The president's assassin, John Wilkes Booth, had entered the presidential box at Ford's Theatre and shot him in the back of the head at 10:15 p.m. as the president watched a play. The commander in chief lost consciousness and never regained it, was taken across the street where physicians attended him, and was pronounced dead about nine hours later at 7:22 a.m. Many security experts at the time viewed the assassination as a fluke.

The next president to die in office also died of a gunshot wound. President James A. Garfield, the twentieth president, was shot in 1881, just sixteen years after President Lincoln's assassination. President Garfield had not been surrounded by a security detail and had no guards. He was shot during an in-town movement in Washington, D.C., while waiting at the Baltimore and Potomac Railroad Station. The gunman shot the president in the abdomen on July 2. Multiple exams by doctors—who did not use sterile technique, as proposed at the time by Dr. Joseph Lister—were performed, including by the physician who cared for the president. Officials brought in inventor Alexander Graham Bell, who had equipment to try to locate the bullet. The prevailing theory directed physicians to do all they could to remove the bullet, but in doing so, they inadvertently produced sources of infection. On July 23, the president developed a fever and died on September 19.

As I think about those two gunshot wounds, I doubt that modern medicine could have saved the life of President Lincoln, but it is highly likely that President Garfield would have survived.

At the dawn of the twentieth century, President William McKinley, the nation's twenty-fifth president, visited Buffalo, New York, to see the Pan-American Exposition at the World's Fair during his second term in office. An anarchist approached him on September 6, 1901, and shot him at point-blank range. Of the two shots to his abdomen, one ricocheted off; the other went clean through his stomach. The president survived for a week, but it soon became clear that internal injuries, made worse by infection and overwhelming sepsis, would prove fatal. He became gravely ill on September 13 and died the next day. It's safe to say that modern medicine would have saved his life, too.

President John F. Kennedy, the thirty-fifth president, was a thousand days into his administration when he died of a gunshot wound to the head while visiting Dallas, Texas. He died a few hours after the shooting. He was forty-three years old when he was inaugurated and forty-six when he was killed.

Eight US presidents have died while in office. Some of them might have survived with modern medical techniques and technology, while some clearly would have died anyway. The physician to the president must keep up with ongoing medical innovations in the hope that they might help healthcare providers do their jobs better.

AN EVOLVING INSTITUTION

The role of the physician to the president has been transformed, permanently changed, from what it once was. From a part-time general physician who might have to be summoned in an emergency across state lines to a full-time physician with extensive experience in multiple disciplines who remains perpetually within two minutes of the president, the role looks very little like it did in 1789.

Good medical care is intertwined with advances in medicine. If you think about Woodrow Wilson's stroke in 1919 or Warren G. Harding's heart attack, they would've turned out differently if these men had served as president just a few decades later.

This fact reminds me of two scenes from *Star Trek IV: The Voyage Home* (1986). In the film, members of the starship *Enterprise* have gone back in time from the twenty-third century to the 1980s to save their world.

In the first scene, Doctor McCoy finds an elderly lady waiting in a hospital bed located in a busy corridor. "What's the matter with you?" he asks.

"Kidney dialysis," she replies.

"Dialysis?" McCoy asks, startled. "My God, what is this, the Dark Ages?"

He grabs a pill out of his bag and says to woman, "Here. You swallow that and if you have any problems, just call me."

A little later, as McCoy and his colleagues flee the hospital, they pass the woman again. This time, she's up and rejoicing. She's grown a new kidney.

In the second scene, Doctor McCoy, Captain Kirk, and a new friend force their way into an operating room to save Lieutenant Chekov, who had taken a long fall and lies unconscious in critical condition. McCoy and the twentieth-century doctor in charge have a heated argument. The hospital doctor insists, "A simple evacuation of the expanding epidural hematoma will relieve the pressure."

"My God, man," McCoy replies, "drilling holes in his head's not the answer! The artery must be repaired. Now, put away your butcher knives and let me save this patient before it's too late!"

Kirk forcefully ushers the confused and unwilling hospital medical staff into an adjoining room, then fuses it shut with a hand phaser. As McCoy puts some kind of advanced electronic device on Chekov's forehead, he mutters, "We're dealing with medievalism here. Chemotherapy. Fundoscopic examinations." And then, twenty-two seconds later, Chekov is cured.

We haven't yet caught up to twenty-third century medical miracles, but we're getting there. In the meanwhile, we keep abreast of the technological and procedural advances that characterize our time and seek to use them in the most beneficial way possible.

ADVANCES IN TECHNOLOGY AND PROCEDURES

Sometimes the WHMU gets to test and use the very newest healthcare technology available, especially to determine the best and most practical use for the innovation. This practice has been going on for decades and continues today. Consider a story about one of history's first known cardiac resuscitation code carts.

The Emergency Care Research Institute (ECRI), located about fifteen miles north of Philadelphia, Pennsylvania, was founded in 1968 as a global, independent authority on healthcare technology and safety. The late Dr. Joel Nobel, one of ECRI's early leaders, recalled how cardiopulmonary resuscitation (CPR) was just coming into broad use in the United States around 1963. Initially the procedure required about eight to twelve nurses and doctors and various pieces of equipment, such an EKG cart, a suction machine cart, an oxygen tank, a backboard, a drug tray, and many cables. Despite the technique's utility, it created a lot of chaos and pandemonium. Dr. Nobel thought, *There just has to be a better way.*

In time, Dr. Nobel developed the MAX cart, which remained on display in ECRI's foyer for years. The MAX cart reduced the required number of team members to three or four and shortened the time to complete its cardiopulmonary support measures to about one minute. Approximately six hundred units were built in the US; one of them ended up aboard Air Force One.

I once spoke to an older butler at the White House who remembered having a MAX cart at the Executive Mansion, but he didn't know where it might have been stored. *Life* magazine ran a feature on modern medical marvels in its January 28, 1966 issue and told how the MAX cart was saving lives. I have been told that a restored MAX cart has been accepted by the Smithsonian Museum in Washington, D.C. I've also seen a sixteen-millimeter training film from the 1960s titled *This Is MAX*, provided to each healthcare system that used the equipment.

Adding to that kind of history, we used several pieces of one-of-a-kind advanced medical equipment to amp up the White House, President Bush's Prairie Chapel Ranch, Camp David, and Air Force One. We had a mobile x-ray machine that fit in two suitcases, for example. We also had the LSTAT, a stretcher-based intensive care unit developed by the US Army.[8] The capability to shoot an extremity x-ray in a trailer or move a critical care patient in an austere environment were important elements to have in a comprehensive plan.

As technology continues to advance, so too will the role of the physician to the president. What will it look like a decade from now? In two decades? In a hundred years? Will there be a Doctor McCoy at the White House in the twenty-third century? While we can only guess what conditions will be like even a few years into the future, one thing is likely to remain the same: presidents and national leaders will continue to need access to trusted, competent physicians. The doctor/patient relationship is here to stay.

That is why every US president, from George Washington's era to the current day, has sought medical advice from trusted civilian and/or military physicians, whether assigned or of their choosing. The president *must* stay healthy, alert, and fully able to carry out the massive duties incumbent upon that office—and the physician to the president plays a key role in making sure that happens.

2

THE CURRENT STATE OF
WHITE HOUSE MEDICINE

If George Washington were to walk into the White House today, it is highly unlikely he would recognize most of what goes on there (except for his own portrait hanging on the wall). With the passage of time, most things change, whether one has in mind medicine, technology, transportation, politics, or nearly anything else associated with humans.

That is certainly true regarding the practice of medicine at the White House and on the Eighteen Acres. In fact, the White House Medical Unit probably has seen more change in how it operates over the past two decades than observers had witnessed in the entire history of the United States before then.

THE WHITE HOUSE MEDICAL UNIT

The primary mission of the WHMU is to provide worldwide emergency action response and comprehensive medical care to the president, vice president, and their families. The secondary mission is to ensure the continuity of the office of the president through life-saving medical intervention and emergency actions, as well as to advise on the implementation of the Twenty-Fifth Amendment of the Constitution. The continuity of the office of the president (COP) makes it clear that the physician to the president has a responsibility not only to the individual but also to the office of the president itself. The most common intrinsic threat is an out-of-hospital cardiac arrest, while potentially the most dangerous threat occurs while providing care under fire, whether gunshots or other types of attack.

The three largest branches of the military (army, navy, and air force) provide active-duty physicians for the WHMU, board certified and experienced in family, emergency, or internal medicine. The surgeon general and the chief of personnel of each service nominate candidates who meet the criteria identified by the director of the WHMU. The process is vetted by the Department of Defense's White House Liaison Office and the Office of the Secretary of Defense (Executive Secretary), all being coordinated by the White House Military Office.

The president of the United States selects a civilian or military physician to serve as the physician to the president. This individual is a White House commissioned officer of the Executive Office of the President responsible for the personal healthcare of the president and the First Family.

After the president selects his or her personal physician, the physician to the president, with the consensus of the director of the White House Military Office and the deputy chief of staff for operations, appoints a military physician to serve as the physician to the White House. This individual typically serves as the director of the WHMU, responsible for medical emergency action and the continuity of the office of the president.

The physician to the president provides medical direction and guidance for the WHMU, with operational oversight by the director of the WHMU. At times, the same person covers both roles, at least for some period. Such was the case with me. I served as both the physician to the president and as the director of the WHMU until

2011 when I appointed Ronny Jackson to be the new director after he was promoted to US Navy captain. Ronny had worked hard as a White House physician for five years, was a competent emergency medicine physician, and got along well with many staffers and Secret Service agents.

Personnel serving in the WHMU are provided by the US Air Force, Army, Coast Guard, and Navy. Each military service normally provides two physicians, two physician assistants, two critical care nurses, one medic or corpsman, one healthcare administrator, and the executive or staff assistants from government service staffing.

The physician to the president also has a responsibility to permanently transform the role as the times may demand. In my case, that meant moving trauma care to the top of the list to be able to stabilize, transport, and provide care under fire. This did not diminish, of course, our ability to manage chronic disease and make prevention a priority, making sure cancer screenings and immunizations were up to date, along with evidence-based recommendations by experts such as the US Preventive Services Task Force.

Every day, acute illnesses or injuries had to be assessed and treated. We gave individuals health advice. While we didn't do true VIP or concierge care, we provided private, secure care with access to specialists that fit into the schedule of the president or the eligible senior staff. First as a member of the WHMU and later as the physician to the president, I tried hard to model the care that the WHMU provided to the president, the First Family, and all staff. I based my approach to the role on the principles of patient-centered medical care.

DUTIES OF THE PHYSICIAN TO THE PRESIDENT

Throughout history, the titles of "physician to the president," "White House physician," "physician to the White House," and "director of the White House Medical Unit" have been interchanged, sometimes used to identify one or even two individuals. The term "assistant White House physician" was commonly used until 1980; it referred to military physicians assigned to White House duties but not in charge of them.

My unchanging personal goals as the physician to the president were to respect patient privacy and maintain strict confidentiality, while at the same time providing access to top-quality care that fit into the schedule of both the president and the First Family. I also had my personal mantra: "No politics, no policy, just trusted medical advice." I promised each of the presidents I served that I would never betray their healthcare privacy or their personal privacy, a promise that I strive to keep even in this book.

The physician to the president has vast responsibility in at least four areas:

1. To coordinate care for the president and First Family.
2. To oversee care for the vice president and his or her family, senior staff, and cabinet members.
3. To direct the WHMU in its emergency actions as an operational unit of the White House Military Office, integrated with the Secret Service.
4. To oversee force protection, population health, workplace health, and safety programs for all workers and guests on the White House complex, including the Executive Office of the President, the United States Secret Service, and the White House Military Office. Each of these latter three groups accounted for about a third of the day-to-day workers on the Eighteen Acres.

As noted in point two, the physician to the president has the oversight and ultimate responsibility for the care of the vice president and his or her family. In February 2009, I appointed Lieutenant Colonel Kevin O'Connor to serve formally in the newly created position of physician to the vice president. Dr. O'Connor was an experienced family physician and had spent tours of duty with the Special Forces, where he had become a leader in combat casualty care.

During my nearly thirteen years at the White House, at least a million visitors toured the Executive Mansion every year, and *every day* somebody had a medical emergency while on the Eighteen Acres. We would provide on-site medical expertise to assist the Secret Service with responding to those situations.

The ultimate job of White House physicians and nurses is to keep the blood in the body and get its patients—presidents, members of the First Family, and those who help the president carry out the chief executive's duties—to definitive care. A multitude of plans remain in place to accomplish that.

THE CURRENT STATE OF WHITE HOUSE MEDICINE

In the past century, the physician permanently assigned to the White House was often thought of as someone who took care of illness or injury for the president, the First Family, staff, or others who visited or worked at the White House. While that remains true so far as it goes, it doesn't go nearly far enough. Over the past two decades, a great shift has taken place in White House medicine as the role has taken on more responsibilities.

Trauma Care

As the years roll on, more and more roles and responsibilities continue to be added to the physician to the president's job description. The most important recent one may be trauma care. If someone on the Eighteen Acres gets seriously injured, the White House physician's job is to assist the Secret Service—who may have a guard, officer, or agent with basic EMT training—stabilize the individual, provide immediate care, and at times participate in transporting the injured person to an appropriate hospital. If an attack of some type occurs, the White House doctor must be able to provide care under fire.

Trauma care is not only reactive but also proactive. The WHMU must be ready for asymmetrical threats, whether chemical, biological, or radiologic/nuclear events.

Preventive Care

Nearly as important in today's world is prevention, whether that means staying up to date on routine immunizations or making sure that travel-related shots or medications specific to a destination or a known public health threat are fully in play. White House physicians must follow evidence-based practices regarding preventive services (whether primary or secondary), especially for screenings of cancer, heart disease, or diabetes. In the past two decades, the focus on preventative healthcare has shifted from illness care alone to include fitness and peak performance.

Acute Care

Doctors must be prepared to deal with unexpected illnesses or injuries, such as an upper or lower respiratory infection, bronchitis, pneumonia, or something similar. Abdominal pain that affects the gastrointestinal tract, including symptoms of nausea, vomiting, diarrhea, or constipation, must receive informed and expert care. Musculoskeletal harm from acute or chronic injuries or overuse must be expertly diagnosed and treated. Whatever the acute care medical issue may be, the physician to the president and his or her staff must be ready to effectively deal with it.

The number one concern is preventing cardiac death. According to the American Heart Association (2008), victims' chances of survival decline 7–10 percent with every minute that passes without CPR and defibrillation. The WHMU, therefore, makes sure that it always has one ACLS-trained biphasic AED healthcare professional within two minutes of the president. This individual must be able to respond, deliver the required shocks, start CPR, and activate EMS. Proximity to the president during work and play, whether home or away, is not optional; it's paramount to what the WHMU does. Sometimes this can lead to overnight stays at places like Buckingham Palace, while at other times it means holing up in far more austere environments.

Occupational Workplace Care

An even newer aspect of expected medical care in the past few decades has been occupational workplace issues—think ergonomics, the chair in the Oval Office, laptops, or computer workstations. Other potential hazards may include noise, exposure to toxicants, or poor indoor air quality. The White House doctor must know something about *all* these issues and must know who can help to give appropriate, discrete evaluation along with expert treatment.

Chronic Disease Management

At the opposite end of the care spectrum is good, old-fashioned chronic disease management of common health conditions such as high blood pressure, lipids, and poor blood sugar levels. And then add to those ailments care for the effects of aging, coronary artery disease, and infections. The contemporary White House physician must be able to manage *all* of this.

CHANGES IN TRAINING

Initial training for the White House medical team took place during the first few weeks of our posting and before long became more robust, standardized, and formal.

When I joined the WHMU, the White House was in a state of transition as George W. Bush was preparing to enter the Oval Office. Very quickly, we worked as a team to remake the OEOB clinic into a worksite injury and illness location to better meet the needs of the office as we moved into the twenty-first century. We would prescribe medications to be filled at military treatment facilities for TRICARE-eligible beneficiaries who worked on the Eighteen Acres. The medications would be delivered via the daily courier run for next-day pickup. As part of a federal workplace, we provided an initial evaluation of injuries or illness for federal employees (military, Secret Service, or staff) who had a White House badge, following federal regulations and legal guidance from the White House Military Office lawyer and White House counsel. We could initiate medications from a modest list of pre-packaged medications and order lab or x-rays with the support of Bethesda Naval Hospital.

Every member of the WHMU received training in basic life support, advanced cardiac life support, pediatric advanced life support, and trauma life support. We also trained in the medical effects of chemical and biological casualties of ionizing radiation, received operational emergency medical training, and completed a trauma training center rotation through a Department of Defense–sponsored trauma training site.

Many of us, more than one hundred since 2007, went through trauma training and EMS ride-alongs at Jackson Memorial Hospital under the guidance of our trauma advisor, Dr. Lou Pizano, a leading trauma surgeon at the Ryder Trauma Center and professor from the University of Miami who directs the Trauma/Surgical Critical Care Fellowship training and serves as chief and medical director for the world-renowned Miami Burn Center. Other WHMU members trained at Shock Trauma in Baltimore, part of the University of Maryland Medical System, or at the University of Cincinnati. Sometimes members would test out through the National Registry of EMTs in association with the state of Maryland (following its requirements). We also utilized a trauma simulation center and had the opportunity to complete EMS training shifts and emergency department shifts.

Afterward, for the remainder of our assignment at the White House, we needed to have sustainment training that would help us maintain our credentials and certifications. Some members continued with EMS or ED shifts, or alternately with the trauma simulation center. Some participated in a tactical medicine course. We set up various cadaver live tissue training sessions with military special operations during a field training course at the FBI Academy or Mayo Clinic in Scottsdale and had a chance to do live intubations in an operating room. Still others participated in a "difficult airway" course.

All of us had a chance to be part of several "assault on the president" (AOP) training exercises conducted with the Secret Service. These usually took place in Beltsville, Maryland, but at times we did the training at Camp David or other locations. Scenarios would involve protective details, military aides, and protective medical teams from WHMU who would go through motorcade, hotel, helicopter, or fixed-wing situations under simulated attacks from teams armed with paintball equipment or other simulated ammunition and weapons. They all ended up in medical situations putting the physician and nurse to work.

We had other training opportunities with the Special Operations Division of the Secret Service; we referred to the Hazardous Agent Mitigation Medical Emergency Response Team as the HAMMER team. We did additional training with the air force's Critical Care Air Transport Team (CCATT) course.

Such training would prepare us for traditional threats of penetrating (guns and knives) or blunt (falls and vehicular) trauma, as well as asymmetrical threats of biological or chemical attacks.

PRESIDENTIAL HEALTHCARE

The physician to the president also must deal with the dichotomy of authorizing primary care physicians to do everything they're trained to do without taking shortcuts, while at the same time keeping specialists from doing everything they're trained to do and instead honing it down only to what's indicated. When medical personnel care for the president or other VIPs, some tend to cut corners while others go overboard.

It takes a lot of time and energy for the physician to the president to arrange access to specialists within a framework that fits the president's schedule and location. The Agency for Healthcare Research and Quality has developed a concept of patient-centered care that has been adopted by those providing care to the president. It is relationship-based and offers whole person, comprehensive care including prevention, wellness, acute care, chronic care, and coordinated care across all elements. It aims to provide superb access to care with short or nonexistent wait times, effective use of state-of-the-art information technology, and an evidence-based, systems approach to quality and safety that utilizes clinical decision support tools and shared decision-making.

So, is this "VIP care"? No, at least not as the term is normally defined. A Very Important Person is typically pictured as someone who stands out and who therefore is given special treatment. In today's world, a VIP might be a high-net-worth individual, celebrity, rock star, or government/political leader.

The paradox of VIP healthcare is that those assumed to have the best access to healthcare often receive the worst. The list of examples here is both long and tragic. Consider, for example, Michael Jackson, "the King of Pop," and Steve Jobs, formerly one of the world's wealthiest men. Jackson's physician complied with Jackson's request for propofol out of his scope of practice and possibly against his better judgment due to Jackson's VIP status. Jobs self-managed his cancer and delayed evidence-based treatment, a practice which is also rampant in VIP care. Both might still be alive today had they not fallen either for VIP care or self-care. Throughout history, a plethora of world leaders and US presidents have received suboptimal care, even though a president is the ultimate VIP, with power, privilege, public recognizability, and lack of personal privacy. "A physician who treats himself has a fool for a patient," declared Sir William Osler. I think it's equally true that "a president who treats himself has a fool for a patient."

During my time at the White House, I advocated for "private, secure care that fits into their schedule," *not* VIP care. When a recognizable public figure receives medical care, it can be disruptive to others in the facility. When physicians and nurses treat their special patients in keeping with their training and experience and not as "big shots"—that is, they follow trauma protocols in a trauma center, for example—those patients have the best chance to receive a standard of care and good outcomes. But when physicians and nurses cut corners because they feel intimidated or have wrong assumptions about what is expected, that is a prescription for failure and poor outcomes. The practice of medicine is built on good information and a solid working relationship based in mutual trust, not friendship. Sound medical advice and mutual respect are both key.

SO, IS ALL OF THIS FREE?

People often think that the president gets free healthcare. That's not accurate.

The president is a federal employee whose annual salary has remained at $400,000 since 2001. As a federal employee, the president has a health benefits plan and can pick from the same list of options offered to US senators and representatives. The president has an enrollment period and pays health premiums just like every other federal employee. The bills may go directly to an accountant, but the process is both private and secure. Presidents can choose to have a dental plan or an optometry plan, both of which are supplemental and optional.

A budget for day-to-day operations is funded by Navy Medicine. Clinical privileges for physicians and medical leadership positions at the White House are maintained at Walter Reed National Military Medical Center, located in Bethesda, Maryland. The commander is the privileging authority. The presidential suite for healthcare is located at Walter Reed, while military oversight and liaising with the Department of Defense is through the director of the White House Military Office. Administrative oversight is through the deputy chief of staff for operations for the White House and the Executive Office of the President.

TRUSTED MEDICAL ADVICE

As previously stated, the overarching mission of the WHMU is to provide worldwide emergency action response and comprehensive medical care to the president, vice president, and their families. At the same time, the WHMU exists to ensure the continuity of the office of the president through life-saving medical interdiction and emergency actions, and to provide medical advice when requested on the implementation of the Twenty-Fifth Amendment of the Constitution.

In whatever ways technology, processes, or various approaches to medicine may advance in years to come, one thing will never change: the physician to the president must *always* provide trusted medical advice. That counsel may cover a variety of medical conditions, whether given to the president, to staff members, to employees working at the White House, or to guests temporarily visiting the Eighteen Acres. The doctor must always remain a source of trusted medical advice for *anyone* needing care or for their loved ones.

Again, the White House doctor doesn't function as a luxury provider or give VIP care. The physician to the president delivers private and secure care that fits the schedule of the busy individuals on the Eighteen Acres who need it and, when appropriate, coordinates and provides appropriate access to medical specialists.

In my view, you might say that the White House medical staff does its best work when the public doesn't even know they're there.

3

PREPARING (UNKNOWINGLY) FOR THE PRESIDENTS

What track does one follow to become the physician to the president? I doubt that any official trajectory for the job exists, but if it does, I certainly didn't follow it.

I grew up near Chattanooga, Tennessee, as the second of eight children. I graduated from high school in 1981 and then attended what formerly was called Southern Missionary College (now Southern Adventist University), affiliated with the Seventh-day Adventist Church, just like my current employer, AdventHealth. At age eighty-four, my father still teaches physics there (and yes, I did take physics classes and labs from him).

For some reason, like Alexander Hamilton, I was in a great hurry. I finished my bachelor's degree in twenty-four months. At the ripe old age of nineteen, I took the Medical College Admission Test (MCAT) and scored well enough to get into medical school. I was Doogie Howser six years before the medical sitcom aired. Loma Linda University School of Medicine in Loma Linda, California, accepted my application, but at the time, it was the third most expensive medical school in the country. Since the school offered no other scholarships, I chose to seek a military scholarship. But which branch of the armed forces should I select?

"Army?" I asked my young and naïve self. *I don't want to go to any army bases. I don't want to wind up landlocked in the middle of nowhere.* So, maybe the air force? "The air force is just a country club," I jokingly told myself. Well, then, what did that leave? The navy! *I'll choose the navy*, I thought, *because I'll be on the ocean. I'll be in San Diego, San Francisco, or Florida.*

I had no idea that the US Navy, in addition to providing care for its sailors worldwide, also takes care of the men and women of the Marine Corps—and there are more than a few marine bases scattered around the globe (as of 2023, twenty-one marine bases operate in the US and eighteen operate overseas).

Despite my naïveté, the die had been cast. I attended Loma Linda from 1983 to 1987 on a US Navy health professions scholarship, which meant I'd have to spend a few years after my graduation taking care of sailors, marines, and their families.

WHOLE PERSON CARE

While at Loma Linda, I learned about "whole person care," which sees how body, mind, and spirit are inextricably intertwined. We learned from thought-provoking physician leaders, such as Dr. Jack Provoncha and Dr. Harvey Elder, who taught and lived whole person care. We also had a theologian with the heart of a clinician, Dr. Will Alexander, who further developed for us the concept of whole person care. They all taught us to use our humanity as an integral part of our medical practice.

Loma Linda is a faith-based medical school, one of the few remaining in the US, so the school also taught us about spirituality. I later came to learn that "spirit" involves more than religion. While spirituality and having a belief system are important, other types of "spirit" also exist, such as team spirit, the human spirit, the Olympic spirit, and the patriotic spirit. When my instructors spoke about "spirit," they had in mind all those varieties. Spirit is separate but intertwined with mental well-being, physical health, and fitness.

During one academic unit of whole person care, our instructors directed us to leave our ivory tower to meet with actual patients. "Put on your white jackets," they said, "and get to know your patient as a person. Don't approach her simply as a fifty-three-year-old woman with gastric cancer waiting for you in room seven. Get to get to know her as an individual. What is her story? What does her story have to do with the disease afflicting her body? How would you characterize her mental state? How are her body and mind and human spirit all acting together?"

As I walked into the hospital room to meet the patient assigned to me, I remember that she looked okay. She seemed about the same age as my mother. I found her staring out the window, and after I introduced myself as a medical student, I told her we were learning about whole person care. I explained that I wanted to know about *her*.

She seemed *much* more excited to talk about her life story than she was about the disease attacking her. But eventually she did reveal her devastating cancer diagnosis. And then she made a statement that I'll never forget.

"You know," she said, "I was living a great life and I always thought there would be more. But for me, there won't be."

She spoke about her two daughters, who were just starting their adult lives. She doubted that she would be there when they got married, when they had children, and when they matured through life. She had thought there would be more . . . but for her, there wouldn't be.

As physicians, we might have been able to slow down the progression of her disease. Perhaps we could even help her adapt mentally to her devastating health news. But we also had to figure out how to bolster her spirits. How could we help her find the peace and healing that she would need to get through the next few days, and then address the shattering issues pressing on both her and her family?

That's when I first clearly saw the critical importance of whole person care. The perspective has never left me.

In medical school, students feel consumed with drinking out of the fire hose of medical information so they can pass parts one, two, and three of their national boards, which will qualify them for a medical license. During their residency, they work hard to become practicing physicians and master their specialty, and then eventually to pass those additional board certifications. They have no choice but to consume an enormous body of knowledge—but too often they skimp on whole person care.

My experience in medical school, and especially with my seriously ill "practice patient," taught me to pay close attention not only to the body, but also to the mind and spirit.

On to the High Desert

After I graduated from Loma Linda, the navy selected me for a program called Physicians and Residents in Medical Universities and Schools (PRIMUS). I completed a three-year family practice residency at Loma Linda University Medical Center. During my last year there, in the fall of 1989 and spring of 1990, I served as the first chief resident of the new residency program.

I finished my first residency in the summer of 1990 and reported for active duty on July 24. The navy sent me to Twentynine Palms, affectionately known as "the Stumps." It's the world's largest Marine Corps base, located in the high Mojave Desert.

For one year I worked at the navy hospital and delivered babies, bringing hundreds of newborns into this world. I also admitted patients of all ages, saw a full panel of primary care patients, and worked in the emergency department, which in that remote part of the country is an indispensable frontline of healthcare.

Crotalus scutulatus, more commonly known as the Mojave green rattlesnake, likes living in the high desert, including around Twentynine Palms. This snake has some of the most toxic venom in the Americas;

a lethal dose is just ten to fifteen milligrams. Its venom affects both the nervous system/brain and organic tissue, including the muscles. The snake typically grows to over three feet long, with some specimens reaching up to four and a half feet. Fortunately, a quick medical response to its bite brings highly successful results, meaning that very few victims die from an attack. I worked at Twentynine Palms in an era before the CroFab antivenin was invented (it was approved by the FDA in 2000), and while our treatment saved lives, it also gave patients horrible serum sickness. Still, all the patients I treated lived and recovered in a couple of weeks. I still have the Polaroids of dead snakes brought in by the victims' families.

Just nine days after I arrived at Twentynine Palms, the forces of Saddam Hussein invaded Kuwait. It seemed to me that the US military sent *everybody* there. I was supposed to go on a mobilization billet three times, but the reservists brought up by the navy all said, "We don't do family medicine. We run weight loss clinics in Las Vegas," or other clinical activities not current with full spectrum care. They all got sent to the Middle East as general medical officers while I stayed behind in the Mojave Desert at a critical, isolated, continental United States (ICONUS) billet.

ACUTE CARE IN HAWAII

After one year at Twentynine Palms, I decided to get married. The navy offered me Subic Bay, Okinawa, Yokosuka, Guam, or Hawaii as my next stop. My newlywed wife, Sandy, advised the latter. Shortly thereafter, I received orders to report to Pearl Harbor at the navy medical clinic.

Sandy and I spent three wonderful years on Oahu, where we began having children. I've always thought it was good for us to be three thousand miles away from family and friends in a place where we had to sink or swim on our own. It didn't hurt, of course, that we did so in balmy, eighty-degree weather, surrounded by beautiful beaches and shimmering blue water.

My first assignment was to run a freestanding emergency room near the Makalapa Gate. We called it "acute care" and had ambulances staffed with emergency medical services personnel. I covered the second shift from 2:00 to 10:00 p.m., as that felt the most exciting.

One night, Sandy picked me up at closing. When we drove out the gate, we noticed a man lying in the road. I stopped and determined he had no pulse. I yelled to my fellow staff exiting the base in other cars to get some equipment. I started CPR. The navy corpsman, who later went to SEAL team training, ran at full speed with a defibrillator and trauma kit. We shocked the man's heart until it restarted and rushed him to Pali Momi Medical Center.

I learned about hurricanes on September 11, 1992. I was assigned to be the medical officer at Camp Smith, a marine command near Halawa Heights, built on the site of a former navy hospital. I was staying there as the sole medical provider with my eight-months-pregnant wife and our beloved pug when Hurricane Iniki rolled through the nearby island of Kauai with Category 4 force, the most powerful hurricane to ever hit Hawaii. Steven Spielberg was there in the last days of filming *Jurassic Park*. We later saw nature's devastating power firsthand. I learned that hurricanes and other disasters required contingency planning and being prepared to provide medical care in unique environments.

I should have known September 11 meant trouble.

At the end of my tour in Hawaii, I had an opportunity to transition from active duty. I strongly considered civilian life in Florida, maybe landing a teaching job at a good hospital. But the navy had another adventure for us.

My superiors selected me for six months of flight surgeon training school at the Naval Aerospace Medical Institute, located at Naval Air Station in Pensacola, Florida, the "home of the Blue Angels." I completed that assignment in mid-1994, and then the navy said, "You're going to London"—and they didn't mean London, Kentucky.

And so, off we went to the United Kingdom.

LEARNING IN LONDON

We remained in England for more than three years, something my Anglophile wife loved. During that time, we saw Princess Diana driving her sports car through Chelsea Harbor, attended book events with Sarah Ferguson, supported Prince Charles and his Prince's Trust event, celebrated the queen's birthday at the Trooping the Colour, and donned our morning dress for our annual soirée to the Royal Enclosure at Royal Ascot, as the queen and Princess Margaret would watch their horses compete. To paraphrase Samuel Johnson, those who tire of London have grown tired of life.

The best part of an assignment overseas, of course, is learning the culture and the people. We chose to "live on the economy" as opposed to military-provided housing. We made lifelong friends with the Barham family; Peter and Jeannie Hudson (a Yeoman Warder ["Beefeater"] at Her Majesty's Tower of London); and a retired brigadier named Scotty Flink, a friend of the ambassador to the Court of St. James's, Admiral William Crowe. I was able to provide flag-level medical care to General Flink and the ambassador's family, along with the admirals stationed in London.

I served as the flight surgeon for Naval Forces Europe at the US Navy medical clinic, with medical offices in the embassy at Grosvenor Square, the navy annex at Seven North Audley Street, and at RAF (Royal Air Force) West Ruislip. In addition to functioning as a flight surgeon, I also served as a family physician for active-duty military, retirees, and their families.

In the military, "collateral duties" are things you're told not to volunteer for because they sometimes consume a substantial part of your life. One collateral duty for me was being assigned to serve as the UK prison medical officer. While I didn't know what the job entailed, I soon discovered that US military personnel—sailors, marines, airmen, soldiers—sometimes commit crimes while stationed in or visiting the United Kingdom. If convicted, they sometimes land in a UK prison.

From that period, I recall a politically incorrect, stereotypical joke about UK prisons. It went like this: "You know you're in heaven when you have an Englishman as your prison officer, a German as your mechanic, and an Italian as your chef. You know that you're in hell when you have an Englishman as your chef, an Italian as your mechanic, and a German as your prison officer."

To learn what a prison medical officer does, I began taking semi-annual visits to the handful of US military personnel in the UK prison system. My basic role turned out to be a well-being check. I didn't need to examine our incarcerated servicemen regarding their physical condition; I could usually tell *that* just by looking at them and asking basic questions. Instead, I focused on trying to ascertain their mental well-being and the spirit they displayed. I also would ask them what made them tick and what brought them joy.

I met one twenty-year-old, straight from the bayou in Louisiana, who suffered from culture shock (in addition to prison shock). He was into sports, so on subsequent visits, I brought stacks of *Sports Illustrated* magazines, either from my personal stash or from the base. You would have thought he had won the lottery. I once inquired about his shoe size since I'd seen that he had only worn-out, basic shoes. I went to the base exchange and bought him some Nike's. Receiving those coveted shoes *really* prompted his jubilation! While I'm not sure I did anything to heal his body, I certainly managed to lift his spirits and deliver a bit of whole person care.

By the summer of 1997, once again I had a projected rotation date (PRD in military lingo), which re-opened the opportunity to transition to civilian life. Once again, we dreamed of getting a family and professional life in the South, maybe at a great hospital in Florida. But once more, the navy had other plans.

"No," they said, "you're going to Quantico, the crossroads of the Marine Corps." *Semper fidelis, semper progredi.* Always faithful, always forward.

And so we went.

YOU CAN SEE THE PRESIDENT FROM THERE

I knew very little about Quantico except what I had learned from watching the 1991 film *The Silence of the Lambs*. The FBI's training academy is located there, west of the interstate. Marine Corps Base Quantico is home to a network of basic, intermediate, and advanced training schools where thousands of marines constantly train. Dozens of tenant commands, as well as marine units stationed near the nation's capital, call Quantico home.

More importantly for my own story, Marine Corps Air Facility (MCAF) Quantico is a secure military airfield on the banks of the Potomac River where Marine Helicopter Squadron One (HMX-1) is located. The H stands for "helicopter," while the M stands for "medium lift." The X originally stood for "experimental," which indicated that any testing in Marine Corps aviation was done there (most testing and evaluation of new aircraft now takes place at VMX-1 in Yuma, Arizona). The 1 stands for the unit's status as an elite squadron.

HMX-1 has become famous primarily because it has served as the helicopter transport for the president of the United States since 1947, as well as for the vice president and other designated VIPs. Its aircraft are referred to as "White Tops," but get the designation "Marine One" when carrying the president or "Nighthawks" when functioning on flights of the Executive Flight Detachment.

This elite squadron has a fleet of White Top helicopters, VH-3D, Sea Knights, and VH-60N Blackhawks (a.k.a. "Whitehawk"), any of which can be deployed worldwide in support of the president's travel. When the president is scheduled to go from point A to point B via helicopter, Marine One provides an "administrative lift" of the president and his immediate family and senior staff to expedite his travel and decrease disrupting the public's travel plans.

If you'd like to get an idea of what a classified mission might look like, I suggest you watch another film, *Independence Day*, which depicts the evacuation of the fictional President Thomas Whitmore.

That'll give you a good mental picture without giving away any classified information. (And no, Marine One does *not* have alien hybrid technology, as some movie fans have wondered).

HMX-1 is located on the Marine Corps Air Facility about thirty miles south of Washington, D.C., where a couple hundred marines, aviators, and aircrew members are stationed. HMX-1 also has another alert facility closer to the White House, on the Anacostia River. During my stint at Quantico, I served as the senior flight surgeon, responsible for the care of the squadron.

My team and I also provided everyday healthcare for eight hundred aircrew who were part of the regular marines stationed at the Marine Corps Air Facility. They were tasked with providing support and air traffic control for the airfield. Every day at such a secured environment, you need a security clearance to pass through various areas of the compound. Our HMX clinic was located behind the fence, on the airfield.

I learned quickly that if you take care of marines, they will take care of you. Quantico had a large navy medical clinic located in the main part of the base. The former navy hospital had become a multi-specialty clinic with full-service ancillary facilities. One day during lunch, an aviator brought in a colleague dripping blood from a laceration suffered during a vigorous game of racquetball. I cleaned up the wound, sewed him up, and got him back to work by 1:00 p.m. He felt extremely grateful for the care and extremely disappointed that earlier he had stopped by the large, modern clinic and been turned away with instructions to "go to the civilian ER in town."

It turned out my patient was the base commander. He picked up the phone, called my commanding officer, and put in some kind words for me.

HMX-1 marines are deployed often and quickly. I made sure their spouses and children were cared for expeditiously, as they often felt frustrated with the complexities of navigating military or civilian medical care. I made more than a few house calls, delivering needed antibiotics to family members. This is the golden rule of healthcare in action: treat others as you would like your family to be treated.

LEAVING AND ARRIVING

Near the end of 2000, the director of the WHMU asked me to come up and eat breakfast with him in the mess located in the basement of the West Wing. Dr. Tubb and I talked mostly about the medical support WHMU and HMX-1 provided the traveling White House staff whenever they went abroad.

He knew that I already had top-secret security clearance, a tough thing to get, and he let me know that there was an opening at the White House—the physician to the president, Rear Admiral Connie Mariano, had announced her retirement with the change of administration. He asked me if I would be interested in moving over to the WHMU.

"Thank you," I said, "but no. You know, my family is happy with where we live. I already have the best job in the navy. You just keep one marine colonel happy, and if you take care of the marines, they'll take care of you."

"Oh," he said, "OK."

Not long afterward, I received a set of orders from the Bureau of Naval Personnel assigning me to the WHMU as a White House physician. I originally came to the White House on a two-year assignment, but soon that was extended.

By the time my job shifted to the White House, my wife and I had two children, ages eight and six years old, both starting elementary school. One had been born in Hawaii and the other in Pensacola during our duty stations there. Despite my new job working on the Eighteen Acres and traveling on official White House business, our family life continued to revolve around supporting our kids in school.

While you might think that our children would express great excitement about their dad working in some capacity with the president of the United States, you would be mistaken. For them, it was just another job—a sentiment that they would express even to the First Couple themselves.

I reported for White House duty in December 2000, right about the time that George W. Bush was certified as the winner of that year's presidential race, defeating Vice President Al Gore. And so, Mr. Bush became the forty-third president of the United States, with Dick Cheney as his vice president. Since I already had the necessary clearance, I just started traveling north on I-95 toward the Washington Monument and the White House instead of south toward Quantico.

And I continued that routine for more than a dozen years, until 2013.

MOVING TO THE WHITE HOUSE

About a decade after Dr. Connie Mariano retired from the navy and as the physician to the president, she wrote a memoir titled *The White House Doctor: My Patients Were Presidents*. For almost eight years, she had been the face of the White House Medical Unit. I learned a lot from her.

Dr. Mariano was a wonderful individual in addition to being a great doctor. She elevated the professionalism and competence of the White House physician even as she helped improve the WHMU as a whole.

But modern medicine never stands still for long. Advances in technology, in procedure, in systems, and in research inevitably alter our idea of "best practices." As the times change, so must healthcare. I saw that truth unfold almost from the first day the White House became my primary place of employment.

I had been uniquely trained and experienced for my new role in that already I had gone on eighteen overseas trips with HMX supporting the White House. I arrived as the junior physician, although my orders from the navy said "White House physician." My first assignment had me working in the OEOB, the medical clinic which essentially functioned as a nurse's station. Medical personnel there did blood pressure checks and provided over-the-counter medicines.

I had just joined the WHMU as a junior White House physician when President Bush took office in January 2001. I had the great privilege of being mentored by Dr. Richard Tubb, an Air Force physician who became a brigadier general. He served as the physician to the president during Mr. Bush's two terms.

Dr. Tubb quickly became the face of the WHMU. I learned a lot from him; he gave me a great deal of helpful professional and personal guidance. He was blessed with great leadership skills and a loyal team, and I felt greatly honored and privileged to do the lion's share of the WHMU's day-to-day work.

As the junior White House physician, I worked primarily at the White House Medical Clinic, located on the first floor of the OEOB. The clinic had operated out of room 105 in that building since the days of President Nixon, who liked to keep a working office essentially right next door. Following federal regulations and legal guidance, we provided worksite care to anyone working on the Eighteen Acres (or to visitors) who had suffered some injury or who came down with an illness on the grounds. The Eighteen Acres, as previously noted, encompasses the White House, the East Wing, the West Wing, the OEOB, the South Lawn, and the North Lawn. We called our services "care by proxy," because we believed that by caring for those who cared for the president, we cared for him.

From my previous navy experience, I was able to bring to the WHMU the electronic medical record system used by all US military healthcare centers whether inside or outside the contiguous United States, , known as the Composite Health Care System (CHCS). For eligible beneficiaries, those in the military or with TRICARE benefits, the system allowed us to order x-rays at a military treatment facility (MTF) and to view results as soon as they became available. We could also order or see results for lab tests and supplement the guidance of the individual's physician. Prescription medications were filled by a pharmacist at an MTF and would arrive on the daily courier run for a qualified individual to pick up if he or she worked on the Eighteen Acres.

Rejoining the WHMU Full Time

I served as the WHMU Assistant Director for Training and Operations from 2001 to 2003. In July 2003, I temporarily left my full-time assignment at the White House to complete a two-year post-doc fellowship and a master of public health degree at Johns Hopkins University. I continued to work part-time serving as the physician overseeing contingency operations at Camp David. I visited Camp David monthly, meeting with the independent duty corpsman and the team of general duty corpsmen to provide oversight.

I rejoined the WHMU full-time as a White House physician in July 2005, and we soon shifted the duties of our physician assistants who had been assigned to the WHMU since 1978. They had provided some coverage to the vice president; now they were fully incorporated into the presidential care team. They also began to serve as tactical medical officers and became involved with our advanced work on sites scheduled for presidential travel.

In January 2007, I became the director of the White House Medical Unit. During that period, we ramped up the care we provided to the president. Critical care nurses traveled with every presidential trip. We were able to formalize the prerequisites and training required to serve as WHMU healthcare personnel. We also standardized the equipment they carried, depending on an individual's role.

In addition, we transformed medical coverage provided for the First Lady of the United States (FLOTUS). The Secret Service requested this change after 9/11, as the FLOTUS is a symbolic national leader. Although FLOTUS involves no continuity of the presidency issues, it is important to have a medical person familiar with her who's able to provide private, secure, top-quality care. The plan, instead of sporadic and by request, shifted to include all US travel. One WHMU healthcare professional would roll with her protective detail, and for overnight trips, would stay at the assigned hotel with the Secret Service and First Lady's staff, ready to respond to medical situations.

BECOMING THE PHYSICIAN TO THE PRESIDENT

After the 2008 election, the physician to the president at that time, Dr. Richard Tubb, intended to leave the White House along with President Bush. So, as the next senior White House physician, I was essentially on deck if I met Mr. Obama's needs and liking.

About two weeks later, after his inauguration, President Obama stopped by my office once more to sign a medical records release.

"I don't really need a doctor," he said to me, "but Michelle and the girls probably do. So, I'm going to go with you." I took that as a great compliment and charge to keep.

That's how I became the physician to the president for the forty-fourth president of the United States, Barack Obama.

ADDITIONAL TRAINING: PREPARATION FOR THE FUTURE

A life of work experience can prepare an individual for crisis. It is no accident that the men and women designated as the White House physician often have extensive military experience. I was no exception.

In addition to my medical training, I completed the Department of Defense's Medical Management of Biological and Chemical Casualties program, which I took at the Aberdeen Proving Ground for the chemical part and Fort Detrick for the biological training portion. In 2001, I learned invaluable lessons from several Homeland Security and Preparedness courses and participated in multiple hands-on exercises with various security councils. From 2003 to 2005, I completed a second residency in occupational medicine and a master's degree in public health (MPH) at Johns Hopkins in Baltimore, Maryland. The instruction I received there, focusing on occupational medicine, the health of workers in the workplace, and public health, was extremely helpful to me. Based on my training and experience as a navy flight surgeon, an FAA aviation medical examiner, the MPH, and other board certifications, I eventually completed board certification in a third specialty: aerospace medicine. My studies in that field helped me a great deal with safety science, anonymous reporting of safety concerns, adverse events, mishap investigation, the person-machine interface, and human factors. In 2009, I interacted professionally with the Centers for Disease Control and Prevention, with their director, epidemiological intelligence service officers, the emergency operation center, and those forward deployed as virologists and global migration experts around the world.

From this brief recap of my medical training, can you see that I didn't choose to specialize in anything? In fact, I ended up as a jack of all trades (and the master of none). All such training helps a physician prepare to effectively serve the president. It also equips the physician to render care to the president's senior staff, key White House personnel, and anyone who works within the very large bubble of the White House.

WHEN IT'S TIME

President Obama successfully ran for reelection in 2012. During those hectic days, I remembered back to 2001, near the beginning of my time at the WHMU. I recalled a talk to staff given by Secretary Andrew Card, President Bush's chief of staff. "You'll know when it's time," he told us.

With the second inauguration of President Obama in the history books, I had accumulated thirty years of naval service, over half of them supporting the White House and the president. I had visited ninety countries. I was blessed to still be married to Sandy, and we had four children, two of them in college and two entering sixth and seventh grades.

Around the middle of that year, AdventHealth in Orlando, Florida, approached me with an offer I couldn't refuse. Would I like to join their physician leadership team? Since Orlando was on my wife's approved list, the answer quickly became, "Florida, here we come."

With my military retirement in July, the role of the physician to the president would transition to the next in line to finish out the administration's term. I felt confident that the people, processes, and platforms I had helped implement would give the president and his staff the best healthcare possible. Dr. Ronny Jackson served as the physician to the president for President Obama and for the first year of President Trump's tenure. Dr. Kevin O'Connor, who I had appointed to be the physician to the vice president, continued to provide exemplary care to Mr. Biden during the failing health and deaths of both his mother and oldest son. Dr. O'Connor retired from army active duty in 2017 but continued to care for the Biden family. Today he serves as the physician to the president for President Joe Biden.

"You'll know when it's time," I'd been told.

I don't remember if I believed Secretary Card's words in the moment, but they certainly proved prescient. After thirty years, I told the navy I wanted to move to Florida, and this time I received no orders to the contrary. They sent me on my way with full retirement benefits, and for the last eleven years, I've had the opportunity and the privilege to use what I learned in the navy and at the White House to help patients, clinicians, and a large national healthcare system become the safest healthcare system in America.

And I still get to live near the water. I guess some dreams of youth do come true.

4

FIVE AND A HALF PRESIDENTS

For more than a dozen years, I served on the White House medical staff directly caring for three US presidents. In fact, however, I can lay claim to meeting five-and-a-half presidents during my career on the Eighteen Acres.

BILL CLINTON'S TRAVEL TEAM

My first assignment providing medical care to the office of the president actually occurred before I even joined the WHMU. In the fall of 1997, I reported to the Marine One helicopter squadron in Quantico, Virginia, at the Marine Corps Air Field (MCAF). For nearly three years, I served as the Marine One flight surgeon, responsible for the medical care of HMX-1, the helicopter squadron that provided the helicopter for the US president whenever he flew in a "White Top" helicopter, the aircraft designated for the president.

Presidents in their second term often try to cement their legacy through foreign policy achievements. President Bill Clinton followed that pattern during his second term when he took eighteen overseas swings.

As part of the training to be part of the helicopter team, you must do "penalty time" flying around, doing a rehearsal, and thus making sure that when the time comes for actual administrative lifts of the president, you're fully qualified and ready to go. During these rehearsals, I often got to sit in the president's chair, called VIP-1, and take in the incredible scenery from that vantage point. VIP-1 faces forward in the helicopter while VIP-2 faces to the rear. The other seats are bench or fold-down jump seats. Every president who has ridden in Marine One has chosen to sit in VIP-1 except President Clinton, who chose VIP-2. He liked to see and interact more easily with everyone in the cabin. (VIP-1 sits in the middle of the cabin with several of the passengers, usually the military aide, doctor, and second protective detail member, behind and out of line of sight.)

Many casual observers considered President Clinton "young and healthy," but all of us on the medical team knew that the *real* President Clinton liked to eat (and not always healthy choices). When he went on a run, it typically was more like a jog for maybe a few laps. He'd frequently stop to chat with people along the way. He's a people person, not a health fanatic.

I had a brief meeting with President Clinton in the Oval Office in January 2001. The experience is vividly imprinted in my mind. He has an incredible personal presence about him, along with the extraordinary ability to focus on you as an individual even though you might never have met. He has a gift to make you feel as though you're the most important person in the world to him at that moment. Even after a short chitchat of only a minute or two, if you meet him again ten years later, he can still remember both you and your conversation. He'll remember everything that was said and will follow up on it. While some may not like his politics or policies, there is no denying that he has an amazing gift for people. I think that's why the American people twice elected him president, an office he held from 1993 to 2001.

One time while at Greg Norman's house in South Florida, the president left the main house to go to a guest house. He stumbled in the dark and tore up his knee. It turned out to be a quadriceps injury, which he had repaired at the National Naval Medical Center in Bethesda by an orthopedic surgeon.

His personal physician, Dr. Connie Mariano, told him, "Somebody with this injury usually gains twenty pounds." Sometimes, under pressure or in a family situation, the injured person buckles down, behaves, and gets in shape. He does what he's supposed to do. That happened this time in the president's case.

A 2013 study published in the *Journal of the American Medical Association* found that the lowest death rates occur among pescatarians—individuals who eat fruits, vegetables, and grains and incorporate fish into their diet, but no other animal products.[9] The next lowest death rate is found among those who eat a vegan diet, followed by lacto-ovo vegetarians. The omnivores, non-vegetarians, have the highest death rate.

Although I wasn't around President Clinton for very long, I knew that you didn't want to embarrass the patients you're taking care of. Still, you are obligated to give them your best advice, whether they take that advice or not. I learned from my experience with President Bill Clinton that to live a healthy life, one ought to regularly exercise and progress to a more heavily plant-based diet.

LENO

Most of us probably love it when friends compare us to some celebrity. I imagine it's fun to hear that you look like Brad Pitt, or Charlize Theron, or Michael B. Jordan, or Zendaya. I get that.

In President Bush's White House, it didn't take long for me to gain a nickname. And somehow, that nickname stuck like glue for both terms of his administration. I suppose that's no surprise since the president himself gave it to me. In fact, his choice proved so popular that most of his staff apparently never even knew my given name. Few of them ever called me "Jeff" or "Dr. Kuhlman." They all knew me by one name only: "Leno."

Now, I'm not a particularly funny guy. I'm certainly no standup comedian. I'm not sure what prompted the president to start calling me Leno, but at the White House, that name became mine for eight years, at least to him and most of his staff.

I discovered later that President Bush has a habit of giving people nicknames. He must have thought I looked like Jay Leno, even though I can't see the resemblance. Whenever the First Lady or the national security advisor would call me Leno, the president would chuckle and feel proud of his nicknaming abilities. In some circles, I guess when you have a nickname, you have arrived.

In any event, that's how I "arrived" at President Bush's White House.

PRESIDENTIAL DIFFERENCES

If President Clinton's schedule said something like, "3:06, do this; 3:10, do that," we all knew that, in fact, such a "schedule" more closely suggested a sequence of events. President Clinton typically did what he wanted to do, when he wanted to do it—a.k.a. "Clinton Standard Time"—regardless of what an official itinerary might say. The president loved to engage with people and have discussions, small and great, which inevitably altered the schedule.

President Bush, by contrast, did pretty much what the schedule announced. If he said something specific should happen at 5:45 p.m., it took place at 5:45 p.m. (or at times, early, which could feel disruptive). We all learned to be ready early, in place, and on time. President Bush was far more punctual than President Clinton.

President Bush also took his health and conditioning far more seriously than did his predecessor. At the time he took office, President Bush was fifty-four years old. If you've read his autobiography, you know that was not always the case.

On the morning after his fortieth birthday, he woke up with a hangover and decided, after having been urged for some time by Mrs. Bush and starting to take his spirituality more seriously, that he would quit drinking. The most important relationship any of us have is probably with our spouse (if we have one). His daughters, Jenna and Barbara, were about two years old at the time.

From that day on, Mr. Bush stopped drinking alcohol. He made an appointment in Dallas, Texas, to meet with Dr. Ken Cooper, the father of aerobics—and he quickly became Dr. Cooper's disciple. In fact, every year until he moved into the White House, Mr. Bush visited the Cooper Clinic.

RUNNING AND BIKING

President Bush ran *a lot* during his first four years in office. When he arrived in the capital, he could run three miles in eighteen minutes and thirty seconds. He was doing *six-minute miles*. Runners will tell you, "That's kicking butt."

The same Secret Service detail that ran with President Clinton also started running with President Bush. All the agents were middle-aged men with a lot of pride and ego. They all said (or thought), "Ah, this is no problem"—and then the president left them in the dust. The Secret Service immediately went out to its field offices to recruit twenty-year-old professional runners who could do five-minute miles.

After those first four years, all that running took its toll on the president's knees. President Bush felt some knee pain from previous meniscus injuries and decided to switch to single-track mountain biking as his primary form of exercise.

As a rule, the president always had to remain in front of the peloton. He would go hard for about an hour to an hour and ten minutes, usually riding close to eighteen miles. That's booking it for technical riders! And of course, unless you crash at least once per ride, you're just not doing it right. You're simply not riding aggressively enough.

The president regularly rode at Beltsville, the Secret Service training center in Maryland, Prairie Chapel Ranch, and Camp David, where trails built for his riding habit ran everywhere. He rode nearly every day, if he could, during the work week at the White House gym or on weekends outdoors, as world events allowed.

Did he ever fall? Of course he fell. Falling off the bike is part of riding the bike, whether you're the president of the United States or a Secret

Service agent sworn to protect him. The WHMU assessed injured riders for their inevitable scrapes, bumps, bruises, and other wounds to make sure none of the injuries were serious; and then we patched up the riders so they could happily go tearing down the path once more.

BIKING AND BRUSH CLEARING AT PRAIRIE CHAPEL RANCH

I estimate that I spent about twelve weeks of my life at Prairie Chapel Ranch in Crawford, Texas, outside of Waco. The Bush family bought the 1,583-acre property in 1999, while Mr. Bush served as the governor of Texas. Before my first visit there, I told myself, "Man, there's nothing pretty in Texas."

I quickly discovered that both the ranch and Crawford are beautiful.

President Bush rode his bike at the ranch, too. Members of the medical team, riding in either a golf cart, a medically equipped all-terrain vehicle (ATV), or a Suburban, would follow the president as he biked. When he crashed, I usually stayed in the vehicle. If he got up and hopped back on the bike, I left him alone. But if he continued to lie on the ground and the agents called out, "Hey doc, we need you," then I hustled out to attend to him.

A couple of times, he suffered leg lacerations. I just wrapped a Coban bandage around the injury and told him, "You're fine." After the ride, we would take more extensive care of the wound.

The president liked that style of treatment. He especially liked that we didn't stop him from getting back on the bike. After a ride on which he injured himself, I'd say, "Why don't you just take a shower and then I'll sew you up?" And that's what we did.

At one point, he got a deep scrape on his chin. I have a few pictures where he also bruised his shoulder; in the photos, you see me examining the non-injured shoulder, too.

I always thought, *If the president of the United States, the leader of the free world, can spend part of a day exercising, then I think all of us can.* You don't have to be a runner or a biker; certainly, President Bush got additional physical activity beyond his two favorite excursions.

In addition to biking, for example, President Bush liked clearing brush on his property. He and his crew would cut down scrub cedar, put it in big piles, and then during the wet season, light it up with flamethrowers. He often made fun of me as we watched the bonfires burn because my hair would always stick up like a hedgehog. Clearing the water-sucking cedar was part of the master conservation plan, allowing the oaks and other natural fauna to grow better. Just before New Year's Day, when it was safe to burn brush, we found ourselves at the end of a canyon with a couple dozen very large piles of brush the size of a building lit up. That canyon became known as "the Twenty-Fifth Amendment Canyon."

Even before the sun rose over the ranch, the president would be back outdoors, either running (during his first term) or biking (during his second). He would return to the house, eat breakfast, and put on work clothes. Then we'd spend many hours clearing the ugly scrub cedar that sucks up water. If you had a chainsaw, you could be a cutter; if you didn't, you became a dragger or a stacker.

After lunch, the president frequently took Barney, his Scottie dog, to go fishing with him on the pond. Our own afternoon activities kept us busy during that time, giving us plenty of opportunities to sew back together various bleeding body parts. I learned from President Bush to lead a physically active life.

WHAT ARE *YOU* STILL DOING HERE?

More than two years after President Bush left office, I accompanied President Obama to the site of the former World Trade Center, destroyed in the 9/11 attacks, to participate in a solemn memorial service. By then, I was serving as the physician to the president.

As we stood there on September 11, 2011, the motorcade of the former president drove up and he got out of his limo—but instead of making a beeline to President Obama, as expected, he approached me.

"Leno," he said, "what are *you* still doing here?"

A decade had passed since the dark days of 9/11, when I'd worked for Mr. Bush in the WHMU. But there I was, still doing essentially the same job, although now serving Mr. Obama as the physician to the president. My former boss simply wouldn't have *dreamed* of letting the opportunity pass without making some good-natured fun of me.

I remember those years fondly, despite my nickname. And by the way, I've met the *real* Jay Leno a couple of times. I've found him to be a wonderful, witty, and charming man.

But I still don't see the resemblance.

THE STAFF LOVED HIM

Many White House staff and ushers have served at the Executive Mansion for what seems like forever. Almost all of them are African American, and *very* proud of their work and heritage in efficiently running the White House. They will gladly point out, "We're actually the ones who built the White House two hundred years ago."

As a rule, staff and ushers personally liked the Clintons. Whenever President Clinton came around, he would personally interact with them—and as already noted, nobody's *ever* been a stranger to Bill Clinton.

But the president they seemed to love the most was number forty-one, George Herbert Walker Bush—and it wasn't hard for me to see why.

When word came that Bush 41 was coming for a visit, the White House long-timers would make sure they were present to show their respect when he walked through the executive residence. "Timberwolf," the former president's Secret Service call sign, would stop and ask each staffer, "Hey, how's your son doing? How's your daughter doing? How's your wife?" President Bush knew *every* person working there and was personally engaged with them—I saw it for myself—and he had lived in the White House only four years. He'd served as vice president for eight years, living at the VP's residence at the Naval Observatory. He and his wife, Barbara, had called that abode their home during the two administrations of President Ronald Reagan.

Because I had many opportunities to take care of President George W. Bush, number forty-three, from 2001 to 2009, I also got to interact with his father a few times when the elder Bush came for a visit, whether at the White House, at Camp David, at Kennebunkport, or at the Prairie Chapel Ranch. Former president Bush would join us for wallyball—volleyball played on a racquetball court—at the Camp David gym, or drive Fidelity, his prized thirty-eight-foot speedboat, as he cruised at extremely high speeds across the Gulf of Maine near Walker's Point, his family home.

During one stay in Wandby, the cabin where support staff stayed on the Bush compound, the Bushes had dinner delivered from Mrs. B's. I passed on the lobster roll but thoroughly enjoyed the sweetest blueberry pie ever, along with homemade vanilla ice cream. I also experienced "speed golf," where the presidents, after attending church service at St. Ann's, would hustle through eighteen holes of golf in less than two hours. No mulligans allowed or needed.

George W. Bush would typically call his father "41," while George H. W. Bush would habitually call his son "43." They consistently used those endearing terms to refer to each other. Occasionally, 41 would jokingly refer to his son as "Quincy," though I don't think the Adams men referred to each other as "2" and "6." President John Adams did live long enough to see his son become president, but he died just over a year into John Quincy Adams's term.

On a few occasions, I had the privilege to meet and to take care of 41. He was in his seventies at the time, but still very active physically and mentally astute.

One time at Camp David, he and former First Lady Barbara Bush came for a visit with their extended family. The former president asked if he could see me for some chronic medical issue that had flared up. "Absolutely," I said.

We met at Eucalyptus, the medical cabin on the compound. I evaluated him, reviewed the care from his physicians both in Kennebunkport and Houston, and was able to prescribe some medication that gave him a bit of instant relief. I informed his primary care doctor in Houston about what we'd done, and then I promptly forgot about the incident. I frankly didn't think much of it at the time; I was just doing the job for which I had been brought to Camp David.

But about a week later, I received in the mail at my home a personal, handwritten note from President George H. W. Bush. He thanked me for the care rendered to him and for coordinating with his other physicians who also were caring for him. In an extraordinary way, he expressed to me his genuine gratitude.

How many VIP patients follow such an example? I suspect very few.

But *many* individuals have stories like mine about the thoughtfulness of George H. W. Bush. From him, I learned to have a positive attitude and a grateful heart.

CHANGE

I first met President-Elect Barack Obama on January 8, 2009, when he came to the White House for a pre-inauguration visit.

His motorcade pulled up by the South Lawn and he walked in through the diplomatic reception room. He took a left by the Map Room. Just beyond the Map Room is the doctor's office, located there since approximately 1901.

That day, President-Elect Obama stuck his head in my office, reached out his hand, and said "Hello, I'm Barack Obama." At this point, he was the most recognizable person on the planet, a forty-seven-year-old meteorically rising in celebrity and popularity. Clearly, on that day, he was still functioning in campaign mode. He didn't appear to realize yet that in twelve days, he would be the president of the United States. The idea simply hadn't sunk in.

"Yes," I smiled and replied, "it's good to meet you."

Humility is a powerful yet rare leadership trait. His humility was a refreshing superpower.

EMPTY NESTERS VS. YOUNG FAMILY

President Bush came into office at age fifty-four. His daughters, Jenna and Barbara, had just graduated from high school; one attended the University of Texas and the other went to Yale. He and his wife Laura were therefore empty nesters, with their schedules to themselves. They also were very familiar with the White House, since the president's father, George H. W. Bush, also had served as president from 1989 through 1993.

Bush 43 would typically rise, be dressed and up before 6:30 a.m., amble over to the Oval Office, arrive there before anybody else, work till midday, go do a workout for an hour, and then return and finish up around 5:00 or 5:30 p.m. That's how he put in his ten- or eleven-hour day.

Things looked very different when President Obama took office. He was forty-seven years old, while the First Lady had turned forty-five just a couple of days before her husband's inauguration. The president and Michelle had ten-year-old Malia and seven-year-old Sasha at home, which made Sasha the youngest child at the White House since JFK's presidency. President Obama also had made a campaign promise to his girls that they could have a dog, so they got a Portuguese water dog as a gift from Senator Ted Kennedy and his family. That's a completely different family dynamic than with President Bush's family.

What do you do when you have two school-aged children? Your home life revolves around school. Everyone in the Obama family would get up by 7:00 a.m. The girls would go to school accompanied by Mrs. Marian Robinson, Michelle's mom, who had her own apartment at the White House. That made the Obamas the first three-generation household in the Executive Mansion in perhaps one hundred years or more (mainly because people in the past didn't live that long).

The First Parents would kiss their girls and send them off to Sidwell Friends School in Bethesda, Maryland. Then, the president and the First Lady often went to the gym on the third floor of the White House to work out with guidance from Cornell, their trainer. They'd mix exercise, ESPN, music, and bonding time.

After that, the president normally took a shower, ate a proper breakfast, walked over to the Oval Office by 10:00 a.m., and didn't leave until 6:30 or 7:00 p.m. He left at that hour so he could be home for dinner, because Michelle had told him, "The girls and I are eating then. If you want to be here for it, then be here." At dinnertime, the family went through their "roses and thorns" routine: "What happened to you today? What was good? What was not so good?" After dinner, the president would carve out time in the evening for extended work.

CHRISTMAS WITH THE VICE PRESIDENT

During my tenure, I had oversight of the medical care given to Vice President Joe Biden, and in early 2009 I appointed Kevin O'Connor as his doctor. I had the opportunity to interact a few times with Mr. Biden during his years as vice president.

One Christmas, he invited me and my family to attend the "friends and family" Christmas party that he and Dr. Jill Biden hosted at the Naval Observatory. I was thoroughly familiar with the official VP residence; I had helped set up the onsite medical contingencies in 2001 when then–Vice President Dick Cheney moved in after an extensive renovation following eight years of Vice President Gore and his large family's stay there. At the Christmas party, my family and I took a holiday photo with the Bidens that they had graciously arranged for us. An hour later, the VP walked up a few steps on the staircase and gave some heartfelt words of thanks and gratitude for the year of taking care of him, along with holiday cheers. He apologized that he and Dr. Biden had to leave the party but encouraged us to enjoy the evening.

He was ready to depart. His motorcade and limo were in position at the front door, but Jill had not responded to his calls out to her.

Without skipping a beat, the vice president scanned the room, saw my attractive and elegant wife, and gently grabbing her hand, he asked, "Want to go to the White House for a party?"

"Let's go," she said, and they proceeded to the departure point. Moments later, Dr. Biden descended the stairs, bid farewell to all, and joined her husband in the limo.

Sadly for my wife, Sandy stayed with me at the Naval Observatory.

DOING THE GINGER ROGERS THING

When I say I've met five and a half presidents, I count Presidents Clinton, George W. Bush, and Barack Obama, as well as having had the privilege of caring for former president George Herbert Walker Bush during his visits to his son, and a few interactions with President Biden when he served as vice president. So, who's the "half president" I've mentioned in jest?

That would be Hillary Clinton.

The media always seemed to portray Mrs. Clinton as difficult, unpleasant, and even a bit nasty at times. But I can testify that whenever I met with her, she was respectful, pleasant, and knew what she was talking about. Policy or politics aside, I would say she was a woman working in a largely man's world (even if such a description rubs some people the wrong way), and in that situation, sometimes you must be a bit tough. You must do the Ginger Rogers and Fred Astaire thing—do it all flawlessly, but backward and in heels.

Whenever she interacted with me about some medical concerns or conditions, mainly on overseas trips, she would consistently listen to what I said, say "thank you," and behave as a model patient.

Mrs. Clinton had received care from Dr. Mariano and the WHMU during the eight years she lived at the White House as the First Lady. She later became a senator from the state of New York. In the 2008 presidential primary, Barack Obama eventually moved past her in a tough contest. But President Obama had such great respect for her that he asked her to serve as his first secretary of state.

US secretaries of state often travel on their own and have a State Department medical doctor travel with them. If they travel with the president on Air Force One, however, which Mrs. Clinton did a few times, then the physician to the president (in this case, myself) provided medical care for all those on board.

On a few instances at overseas locations, Secretary Clinton asked my medical advice for this or that issue. I was able to render it and then help her to communicate directly with the physicians caring for her back home. In *all* my encounters with Secretary Clinton, she was both positive and professional. I felt that she treated me and others around her with respect. In my experience, she was nothing like what some have depicted in various media encounters.

My interactions with Secretary Clinton taught me to judge a person by my own firsthand interactions with the individual and not through reports or accounts that may be distorted with prodigious amounts of spin.

During my dozen years at the White House, I learned that presidents are people. Red or blue, luckily they are the same on the inside. And in caring for them, I learned the valuable life lessons of progressing to a more plant-based diet, living a physically active life, practicing temperance in one's personal habits and choices, and having a heart of gratitude.

PART TWO

———◆———

The Changing Face of
Presidential Healthcare

5

The Transformation of White House Medicine

As stated earlier, I received my medical training at Loma Linda University in the 1980s. One of the first concepts introduced to us by our professors was whole person care. A person is not just a physical body with pathophysiology but an interconnection of mind, body, and spirit.

It's About More than Caring for Bodies

Even in peacetime, doctors must deal with tragic deaths. And when confronting death during a noncombat time, the opportunity always exists to deal not only with the body but also with the mind and the spirit. Even before I got to the White House, I saw the importance of whole person care—and developed protocols to provide care for more than bodies to my charges.

We had many young marines from unstable families who could not provide much support. Some of these marines got into personal relationships a bit over their heads; they lacked the life experience to positively deal with such loaded situations. For example, a marine was in a stressful relationship with a woman much older than he was. One evening during an argument, with access to a handgun, he pointed it under his chin and pulled the trigger. But he had aimed the gun forward just a bit, and whether accidentally or intentionally—to this day we're not sure—the bullet passed almost magically between his optic nerves, sparing his eyesight. The projectile basically went up through his sinuses, exiting his forehead.

To address the spate of suicides we were experiencing, I had enlisted the help of Lieutenant Commander Bob Williams, the navy chaplain assigned to the Marine Corps Air Facility. We also had begun working with Lieutenant Commander Andy Davidson, a licensed clinical psychologist assigned to Marine Barracks Washington. All three of us had top-secret, Yankee White security clearances.

We had already been working together for a year or two assessing marines assigned to presidential duty. Part of our job was to make sure that they had no serious mental health issues. If we discovered they did, we got them the treatment they needed. If they wanted to speak with a chaplain, Lieutenant Commander Williams was wonderful. If they needed cognitive behavior therapy, Dr. Davidson would set up private and secure sessions as a psychologist. If they needed medication—psychotropic medication or other medical intervention—I took care of that. We worked together as a team to treat the whole person.

We dealt appropriately with everyone's security clearance. Sometimes we recommended another assignment if it seemed in the best interest of the military and the individual. Often, though, we could recommend holding the clearance in abeyance; once the individuals had coped with the relevant issues, they could return to their former jobs with clearance intact.

In response to this new challenge of suicidal behavior, we developed a three-tiered approach. We called the first tier "primary prevention." We provided educational materials delivered in the form of town halls where the three of us would do squadron talks. We did this with every individual assigned to the squadron and the air facility.

For the secondary tier, we targeted groups of high-risk individuals. We went to each group toiling under extreme pressure, whether they were involved with travel due to an election campaign or with some other sensitive operation. We had one-hour sessions with those groups in their workspaces or hangar, following a script and presenting targeted information. We also remained attentive to specific individuals who appeared to need help.

For our third tier, we invited any individuals who wanted help to come and talk to us one-on-one. Many individuals accepted our invitation.

Our three-tiered approach seemed to work well, and for the rest of my time at HMX-1, we had no more serious incidents. I consider it yet another example of the power of whole person care. We used a chaplain, a mental health professional, and a physician to address the body, the mind, and the spirit, whether as individuals or as members of a group.

DEATH STILL COMES KNOCKING

Even in the absence of serious behavioral issues, death sometimes still comes knocking. We had one gunnery sergeant who spent three decades in the marines and then retired as a master sergeant (an E-8 in the marines). Tragically, within the next week, he had a heart attack and died.

Many senior marines heard what happened and expressed the common sentiment, "Oh, man, you don't want to retire, because then you die."

A lieutenant commander, a pilot in his forties, transferred to an air facility in South Carolina. He also had a heart attack and died while running.

A third pilot was driving a Miata sports car on a country road in northern Virginia. As he passed another vehicle, he overcorrected and died in a single-vehicle traffic accident.

Perhaps worse were cases when marines died while training or while on routine peacetime exercises. On Sunday morning, April 9, 2000, I received word that one of our V-22 aircrafts had gone down during the night at Marana, Arizona. Its two pilots, Major Brooks Gruber and Lieutenant Colonel John Brow, had died in the mishap, along with seventeen others, all of them active-duty marines.

Our squadron safety officer and I got on the next plane out of Washington Dulles International Airport. We flew to Tucson and immediately visited the scene of the wreckage. I served as the senior officer for the rescue. Unfortunately, we shifted quickly from rescue to recovery of bodies. A small team from the Naval Safety Center also had arrived. Without a chaplain present, I led us in reciting Psalm 23. We truly felt we were in the valley of the shadow of death.

As I looked at the nineteen human corpses melted into the carbon fiber skin of the V-22, I pondered out loud as we worked to sort the remains, "Black, white, red, yellow—we are all the same. We are all equal in death."

An investigation determined that the craft had descended at far too high a rate, causing it to enter a "vortex ring state" in which it lost lift. In midair it flipped on its back and then slammed into the ground, nose first. A two-month moratorium on testing the Osprey immediately went into effect, followed by months of redesign. The aircraft finally entered operational service in 2007.

Two officers who took part in a noncombatant evacuation operation (NEO), but who had safely landed elsewhere, arrived the day after we did to survey the crash site with me. One was Jim Wright (call sign "Lefty"); the other was Lieutenant Colonel Keith Sweeney, the officer in charge of the multi-service operational test team (MOTT). We surveyed the crash site together and completed the initial part of the inquiry until we could turn it over to the formal investigative team.

Tragically, both of those men lost their lives later that year in mid-December, when the V-22 they were flying in North Carolina went down in the woods due to a mechanical failure. News of the mishap and their demise came to our squadron commanding officer, Colonel Mac Reynolds, and I as we were providing Marine One support to President Clinton during the fifty-fourth and final international trip of his two terms in office. During that visit, the president met with Queen Elizabeth II and gave a speech at the University of Warwick after meeting with the prime minister, Tony Blair, in Belfast.

Once again, I talked to the entire deployed squadron and met with a targeted group of pilots and individuals who had known the deceased.

When such tragedies strike, many of those left behind need whole person care. Even in peacetime, we remember that death comes knocking at any hour it chooses. Offering whole person care allows us to do more than just patch up wounded bodies. Without it, some of them will fall into pits from which no traditional medicine can rescue them.

WHOLE PERSON CARE

Because of my many experiences showing the importance of whole person care, when I arrived at the White House Medical Unit, I set up an integrated medicine network featuring four primary components.

The first component focused on mind-body-spirit (not necessarily "spirituality," but the human spirit). We brought in a White House chaplain staffed by the military, as we recognized the important effects of the mind and spirit on the body's proper functioning. We focused on mental health and well-being, not merely on mental illness. We also offered cognitive behavioral therapy, provided by a licensed clinical psychologist who worked either at the marine barracks or at HMX-1. The individual, of course, had the required top-secret clearance.

The second component of the integrated medicine network covered biological-based practices, such as nutrition. We had an outstanding clinical nutritionist from the FDA who periodically came down to the White House. She also spent time in the White House mess, located on the ground floor of the West Wing, where senior staff and their guests can eat breakfast or lunch without leaving the building. She provided healthier options in addition to classic selections.

The third component focused on manipulative (or body-based) practices. We had trained massage therapists who either were vetted or staffed by the WHMU, physical therapists certified in spine manipulation, or WHMU osteopaths current in their clinical competence of osteopathic manipulation.

The fourth component, energy medicine, became very popular. At least one or two White House physicians had gone through formal training in acupuncture and kept up their certification. We provided these treatments, as appropriate, to anyone who lived or worked on the Eighteen Acres.

All four of these components fit into whole person care. I believe it's critical to focus not only on injury or illness but also to give equal attention to mental well-being and strength of spirit.

Sometimes we forget that world events can powerfully affect the spirit of a president, whether those events involve nations on the edge of a nuclear exchange, wars in the Middle East, mass shootings of children in the United States, or US military personnel killed in combat or in peacetime. All such tragic events can take an extreme toll on the comforter in chief, who takes his duties very seriously and with great solemnity.

The most effective way I know to buoy the presidential spirit is to take a whole person approach to healthcare, recognizing that each of us functions best when the body, the mind, and the spirit stay in unison.

One part of our integrated approach to healthcare involved developing one track for the president, while another part concerned those who support the president. To address both areas, I followed the concept of "care by proxy." By taking care of those who cared for the president, we cared for him.

That care had to be made available anywhere, as allowed by regulations, on the Eighteen Acres where employees and staffers worked every day, and within the umbrella of the traveling White House, which means anywhere in the United States or in the world.

KICKING THE SMOKING HABIT

Sometimes, whole person care meant support—and sometimes, it meant some tough love.

President Obama—the portrait of a young, vigorous, healthy male—was a smoker during his first year in the White House. In his books about his life, he wrote that he had started smoking as a teenager. Once in office, he was "95 percent cured," but we all know what that means for a smoker.

I quietly gave him a briefing book containing information about kicking the habit. I would give anyone the same advice I gave to him: "The average smoker quits at least eight times before they succeed. Here are several options to help you quit." He chose the one that he thought would work best for him.

I eliminated one of his sources of the product, and then we persuaded his closest friend, his smoking buddy, to stop at Christmas. The president found himself left all alone.

My private advice was, "You've got everything: fame, fortune, a wife who'll talk to you, kids who love you—but it won't matter, because you'll be dead in a few years from heart disease or cancer."

In the president's physical that I signed that year, I received a lot of grief from the medical community because I had written, "Continue smoking cessation efforts." The more obvious statement would have been "Stop smoking," but I believed that I had to be factual and truthful. Other White House doctors might be willing to say that someone was seven feet tall and weighed a hundred pounds, but I didn't want to mislead the American people.

During President Obama's first Martha's Vineyard working vacation in August 2009, we were sitting on a golf cart, discussing his healthcare and planning for the physical. He told me, "I have learned to never lie to the American people, as they will always find out the truth."

Even before he quit smoking, the president's normal blood pressure and lipid profile gave him an average risk of having a cardiac event (heart attack or death) in the next ten years, with a 7.3 percent chance. But I told him, "If you're a non-smoker—which is zero cigarettes in twelve months, in terms of the Framingham study—you will be able to get down to 2.5 percent." In other respects, he was in excellent physical shape, maintained an ideal weight with a BMI of 23.7, and truly ate a healthy diet.

"I'll quit," he told me, "when the Affordable Care Act is passed." That legislation was passed on March 23, 2010, at which time I sent him a note with a smile: "Okay, you've had your last cigarette."

He stopped on his own a week later, and to my knowledge, he didn't relapse. He continued to occasionally use some Nicorette gum, but just because he liked it. I believe Michelle is the one who announced to the world later that year that he had successfully kicked the habit.

THE SMARTPHONE ERA

The doctor's black bag of past generations has been replaced, first by the cell phone and now by the smartphone. Email, digital imaging, video conferencing, and the web now are all at the fingertips of those who care for the president. Telemedicine is not a novelty but an essential tool that enhances doctor-patient interaction and improves their relationship.

The history of electronic health records at the White House goes back to about 2001, when the clinic in the OEOB first utilized CHCS as part of a Department of Defense initiative aimed at upgrading laboratory, x-ray, and medication services. In 2009, an upgraded system was brought into the doctor's office at the executive residence. This system included records of outpatient encounters within the electronic medical record (EMR). This EMR access extended to the medical annex on board Air Force One, at Camp David, and in an annex clinic at Bolling Air Force Base (covered by WHMU personnel). It grew to include the White House Communications Agency, the Marine Corps Air Facility in Quantico, and contingency locations and remote global sites with internet access. When the military shifted its electronically accessible health records to the Armed Forces Health Longitudinal Technology Application (AHLTA), the WHMU followed suit.

In addition to lab, x-ray, pharmacy, and outpatient notes, other modules kept up immunization records as well as gave access to the most current medical information.

THE KEY: INFORMATION AND RELATIONSHIPS

The practice of medicine comes down to information and relationships. Every healthcare provider must build trust with their patients, who need to feel confident that their doctor or nurse knows what they're talking about and that they care for them. Medical professionals must be able to sift from the vast amount of information available to choose the most current information pertinent to the patient's unique situation.

Chief executive medicine comes with a paradox of expectations and barriers. The leaders we care for expect continuity of full-spectrum care designed specifically for them, whether it's fitness, wellness, dental, traditional injury or illness care, chronic disease management, access to consultants, or appropriate use of complementary and alternative medicine. They expect that we care for their whole selves.

It needs to be seamless. It needs to be orchestrated. It needs to fully respect the patient's medical and personal privacy. It needs to be of the highest quality. And it needs to cross the military, public, and private sectors. In other words, it's the usual healthcare balancing act of quality and access.

At the end of the day, we can't give care if we're not there. Major barriers to personal access exist at the White House. Many want to control health access to the president's time or schedule. Real time limitations also exist when the president's every minute is scheduled. Physicians to the president must work to fit the care they provide into the time limitations given to them—and know when it is appropriate to expand those designated times.

6

FROM ABSENCE OF DISEASE
TO MAXIMIZING FITNESS

For a long time, traditional medicine focused on health as the absence of disease. Although that remains the dictionary definition, it seems to me a very subjective characterization. We know doctors help sick people and those suffering from illness, but today we focus more on health by maximizing fitness. At the White House, therefore, we focused on the concept of fitness in addition to mere health.

Fitness involves taking control of one's personal health through healthier eating, leading a more physically active life, being temperate, and encouraging a positive mental outlook. Good fitness can improve job performance and, almost like a fountain of youth, can add years *and* quality to one's life.

Under the old paradigm that defined health as the absence of disease, White House doctors issued a standard report that included results from a physical exam, some lab data, results from any diagnostic tests, some assessment of certain organ categories, and a judgment about the general condition of the president's body.

I worked hard to change the narrative from health as merely the absence of disease to fitness designed to help us optimize the individual's performance.

Both President Bush and President Obama were physically active and had remarkable fitness, which I think contributed to their ability to do their job. We did several things with both presidents that we never advertised, including treadmill fitness testing with an estimation of VO2 max, gait analysis, body fat analysis using a BodPod, and functional movement screen, which did improve their fitness and hence boost their performance. If you can optimize your physical performance, then you, too, can optimize your human performance.

Better physical fitness improves the mind. Not only do we feel better and have an improved sense of our well-being when we get in good physical shape, but fitness supercharges the mind for optimal performance. Such supercharging can be as simple as getting adequate rest or combating the effects of jet lag (or time zone desynchronization), so long as it's done in a healthy way that avoids clouding the mind.

The third aspect is the spirit: being sensitive to the individual's spiritual beliefs, being sensitive to their patriotic spirit, and being sensitive to their human spirit.

As noted, President Bush was an avid runner when he came into office. At times he would run three miles, and when he pushed it, he could clock in at about eighteen minutes and thirty seconds, close to a six-minute mile.

After many years of pounding on his knees, along with various athletic injuries over time, the president shifted to mountain biking at the beginning of his second administration. Biking puts far less stress on the knees but still gives the cycler a great aerobic workout.

By the time President Obama came into office, he already had gained fame for playing full-court basketball with men much younger than himself. He also took care of himself by eating a good diet. After

JEFFREY KUHLMAN, MD, MPH

a short workout, he then took a shower, ate a proper breakfast (such as eggs and toast), got dressed in business attire, and used the elevator to go down to the ground floor. The doctor's office sits close to the elevator, and so as he'd pass by, at times he'd greet me or say "hi" to the nurse. He'd then walk through the tradesman entrance along the West Colonnade, stroll through the Rose Garden, and enter the Oval Office to begin his day of work.

Exercise and fitness are not only for the president "at home," of course; they're equally important for the frequent times when the president hits the road.

Whenever we traveled together, President Obama started off his day with exercise at the hotel gym, using the treadmill, stationary cycle, and weight training routine written out by his personal trainer. President Bush would do a running or cycling workout as often as possible wherever he was visiting.

No Statutory Medical Requirements Exist

For a presidential candidate or an individual who holds the office of the president, no statutory medical requirements or fitness standards exist, aside from being at least thirty-five years of age.

Many presidents have served with various physical conditions and functional limitations or impairments, whether temporary or permanent. Reasonable accommodation helps such individuals to optimally perform their presidential duties. At the Philadelphia convention in May 1787, the Framers wrote Article II, Section 1 of the US Constitution, speaking of the "inability to discharge the powers and duties of said office." Some have debated the meaning of the word "inability" and whether it refers to a physical condition or a mental or intellectual one.

The Twenty-Fifth Amendment, ratified in 1967 (which we'll shortly consider in more depth), uses the phrase "unable to discharge the powers and duties of his office" in Section 3 when referring to a voluntary transfer, and in Section 4 when addressing involuntary transfer. Senator Birch Bayh, the main author, in his Senate testimony of February 1965, testified that he intended to describe the impairment of a president's faculties if "he is unable to make or communicate his decisions as to his own competency."

In the twenty-first century, the concepts of "critical thinking" and "critical decision-making" have taken center stage. Most, if not all, physical impairments can be accommodated—*except* the ability to think critically, to effectively communicate those thoughts, and to exhibit critical decision-making. Nevertheless, to this point in our history, we have tended to focus far more intently on a president's physical health than on his or her mental acuity. That may be changing (see chapter 11).

FROM ANNUAL PHYSICAL TO PERIODIC CHECKUPS

The public perceives, and the media tends to perpetuate (or even expect), the idea that an "annual physical of the president" must be done and reported to the American public. In fact, no such requirement exists, much less official guidance for such annual exams. Modern medical practice hotly debates both the need for and the performance of an annual physical.[10] Many expert groups recommend against annual preventive examinations in asymptomatic patients. They call the practice "obsolete."

President George W. Bush and his White House physician, Dr. Tubb, typically completed an annual exam at the end of each summer. Results from that physical were reported just before Mr. Bush's month-long working break at his Prairie Chapel Ranch, which coincided with the Congressional summer break.

President Obama had a more evidenced-based, pragmatic approach to healthcare. The two of us discussed the varied elements of the exam while we were at Martha's Vineyard in August 2009 and considered how to use it as an opportunity to perform age-appropriate evaluation. His first periodic physical was performed at Walter Reed National Military Medical Center in Bethesda in February 2010.

During my time in the WHMU, we began utilizing several new approaches to health exams. While I continued to give a routine physical, do some basic diagnostic tests, and perform the exam that has become so familiar to most Americans, I also introduced a new fitness test for the presidents.

Working in conjunction with Dr. Drew Contreras, a physical therapist, we took the president to the DiLorenzo Clinic at the Pentagon, where a physical therapist did a gait analysis as the president walked and then ran on a treadmill.

We also put the chief executive through a functional movement screen (FMS), which analyzes individuals for risk of injury due to any performance-limiting movement pattern. The screen evaluates seven fundamental movement patterns and is intended for those reporting no current complaints of musculoskeletal pain. Many men pride themselves in their strength, but the functional movement screen humbles most of us. It humbles even many athletes because it checks one's core strength—can you plank? Can you balance?—and then identifies deficiencies and targets them over time.

The third part of our fitness assessment took place on a treadmill and assessed for VO2 max, which indicates an individual's level of aerobic conditioning. President Bush had exceptionally high aerobic conditioning when he entered office. His fitness testing, assessing VO2 max, put him in the top 1 to 2 percent for his age range.

The fourth part required participants to get down to their skivvies and enter a BodPod, which directly measures the individual's body fat percentage.

Those four measurements give us a very good assessment of individual fitness. While these assessments weren't part of the customary periodic physical, they did provide basic information for the president (or others) that that they could then choose to use to improve their personal fitness.

It was decided not to release to the public the additional information from those fitness tests, mainly because of the uninformed scrutiny we expected it might generate. We could just hear the questions:

"Why are they focusing on the president's fitness? We just need him to run the country!" Such anticipated objections seemed odd to me, as it seemed (and still does seem) self-evident that a fit president can do a better job of running the country than an out-of-shape one. The president appreciated the additional insights and used the information to improve his own fitness.

The purposes of the periodic exams that I performed and supervised were to provide the public with a candid medical assessment of the president's ability to carry out the duties of his office, both now and for the duration of his tenure, and to provide the president with every opportunity to enjoy the benefits of good health now and for decades to come. The examination focused on evidence-based guidelines tailored to the individual uniqueness of the person and his occupation.

The report on the president's health should reasonably consider personal and patient privacy but must be precisely factual and non-superfluous. Crossing that line may catch the attention of partisans, but such an act poorly serves the patient, the public, and the profession. Straying from the facts can break trust and devastate everyone involved. Words and the meaning of words are important.

Health as traditionally defined is the absence of disease, or to be free from injury or illness. Fitness is the ability to perform tasks with vigor and alertness without fatigue while yet maintaining a reservoir of energy; it involves aerobic conditioning and functional movement capabilities. Wellness encompasses the inextricably related concepts of mind/body/spirit, based on mental, physical, and spiritual components of a whole person.

A medical report typically covers many traditional aspects of health, while assessments of fitness do not typically find their way into that report. For past presidents, the fitness assessment—cardio/respiratory, strength, and flexibility, with normative percentile data specific to their sex and age—was periodically presented to the president and used to create their own personal training program and to track individual progress.

A summary stating that good health is merely the absence of disease or injury fails to address either fitness or wellness, which I believe does the nation a disservice. The statement "fit for duty" is the physician's personal testament to the president's ability to perform the duties required by the Constitution, and it should include both fitness and wellness components. We don't expect our presidents, their physicians, or the press to be perfect, but we do expect them to be truthful.

Unfortunately, not all physician's reports are created equal. The physical exam of President Trump and the briefing in the White House Press Room on January 17, 2018, contained information that was obviously not factual, such as height, weight, and body mass index, and omitted important cardiac testing that was done. Additionally, it included unnecessary superlatives such as the president having "superior genetics" or living "to be two hundred," statements that provided fodder for a *Saturday Night Live* opening skit.

FRAMINGHAM RISK SCORES

The Framingham risk score, a commonly used algorithm in medicine, is used to calculate an individual's risk of having a cardiac event—death or heart attack—in the next decade of life. It is based on the age and sex of the individual and considers several key health risk factors, such as smoking history, cholesterol levels, and blood pressure readings.

Consider the calculated Framingham score for President Clinton when he left office. A copy of his last physical is public record, published in December 2000. When he left office in January 2001, his blood pressure and lipids were under control and his body mass index was reasonable. His Framingham risk score was 7.5 percent, lower than the 10 percent average for his age and sex. He was on a cholesterol-lowering statin, of course, and he didn't smoke cigarettes. When he left office at fifty-four years old, he was in good cardiovascular shape.

Now fast forward about three-and-a-half years. Middle-aged men often stop taking their medication and start eating whatever they want, especially if they don't have their doctor on their back closely monitoring their numbers and providing motivation. They don't prioritize exercise because they get "too busy."

I woke up on September 7, 2004, to a newspaper headline announcing that former President Clinton had successfully undergone emergency heart bypass surgery the day before at NewYork-Presbyterian, part of the Columbia University system. He had undergone a quadruple bypass and was expected to have begun a safe recovery from the four-hour operation. During the surgery, his medical team discovered that some of his arteries were at least 90 percent blocked. Without that surgery, experts said, the former president likely would have suffered a major heart attack within a short time.

How does an individual go from a lower-than-average Framingham score to quadruple bypass surgery, all in less than four years? Part of the issue, many times, is lack of compliance. And while you might think that VIPs get the very best care, many times, they don't.

I've reproduced the results of the first physical we did on President Bush after he arrived in Washington. His Framingham score was 4.9 percent instead of 13 percent (the average for his age and sex). For a fifty-four-year-old, non-smoking male with a total cholesterol of 170, HDL cholesterol of forty-two, and systolic blood pressure of 118, he had a calculated 4.9 percent risk of myocardial infarction or cardiac death in the next ten years—much lower than the average male of his age. More than two decades later, he is alive and well, following the guidance of his physicians and leading a physically active life.

BASKETBALL INJURIES AND COLONOSCOPIES

The increased focus on fitness didn't mean that mundane, routine medical care could be neglected. One Friday after Thanksgiving, President Obama decided to play some basketball. An opposing player unintentionally elbowed him in the mouth (as happens) and he returned to the White House to get it taken care of. I was already at the clinic, seeing another member of the extended family. I had the opportunity to oversee the evaluation of his oral injuries and get him expertly sewn up by a navy surgeon who fortuitously was in my office when the injury occurred.

One of the first extended conversations I had with President Obama took place in January 2009 when he astutely asked me whether he should have a colonoscopy. I told him that he was at normal risk, without a family history of colon cancer. The then-current recommendation from the experts was to get a colonoscopy at age fifty, or at age forty-five for African Americans.

"Perfect," he said with his trademark smile. "I'm half and half, and halfway between forty-five and fifty. I'm forty-seven; let's get it done."

Colorectal cancer screening guidelines had just been updated in 2008 by a joint committee of the US Multi-Society Task Force, a group that included the American Cancer Society, the American College of Radiology, and the American College of Gastroenterology.

The newly published preferred colorectal cancer screening recommendation was to have a colonoscopy every ten years, beginning at age fifty, with screenings to begin at age forty-five for Black people. A computed tomography/colonography every five years was an approved, alternate colorectal cancer prevention test. It carried a grade 1C recommendation. Grade 1 means a strong recommendation in evidence-based medicine lingo. Grade C means the evidence comes from observational or clinical experience, versus the gold standard of randomized controlled studies. The "lower quality evidence studies" still supported the strong recommendation.

A computed tomography scan (or CT colonography) is a non-invasive procedure that takes x-ray images from different angles and then uses computer processing to create cross-sectional images of the body's interior. At the time, the National Naval Medical Center in Bethesda had one of the premier integrated colorectal cancer screening programs in the nation, where they did CT colonography. Bethesda also had two radiologists with subspecialties in the reading of CT colonography. If a polyp showed up on a CT scan, doctors could then move directly to an optical colonoscopy for the removal of the polyp, as they were already prepped.

At the time, only half of the American population that should have been getting colorectal cancer screening was getting the screening done. CT colonography is safer and less invasive than optical colonoscopy and many patients prefer it. One downside to the procedure is that about 10 percent of the time, an incidental finding necessitates further investigation. A big advantage for the president was that he would not have to go under anesthesia for the twenty to thirty minutes it normally takes for the procedure, so he would not have to invoke Section 3 of the Twenty-Fifth Amendment (see chapter 11).

The president asked me to arrange for the CT colonography to be done during his regular periodic physical. With his colon prepped, if doctors found something abnormal, the GI suite was standing by. Screening colonoscopies have about a 5 percent chance of finding a polyp or something abnormal.

President Obama's first periodic physical exam was performed on February 28, 2010, at the National Naval Medical Center. At the same time, he underwent a CT colonography, the first time in history that a virtual colonoscopy had been performed on the president of the United States. Not only did his test provide an example for the rest of the country, but best of all, it also showed no abnormalities.

THE LASTING INFLUENCE OF DR. KEN COOPER

President Bush stated in his autobiography that he began a life of temperance after his wife confronted him about his former wild ways. He soon became a disciple of Dr. Ken Cooper, a leading advocate for the central role of fitness. From that time on, President Bush started putting a great deal of energy and time into exercise and physical fitness.

I had the privilege of meeting Dr. Cooper a few times, learning from him and working with him. At one time, Dr. Cooper had been an air force flight surgeon. He coined the term "aerobics." When I asked him how he developed the idea, he thought back to his pre-med biology days, when his professors discussed bacteria. He learned that bacteria exist in two forms, aerobic and anaerobic. In 1966 he simply took the word "aerobic," an adjective, put an "s" on it, and started using the word as a noun. Two years later, he published his book *Aerobics*, and in 1970 he founded the Cooper Institute, still one of the world's leading research organizations in preventive medicine, exercise science, and obesity.

Dr. Cooper has amassed an extensive collection of data about physical fitness and physical endurance. Over many years, he put hundreds of thousands of individuals on treadmills. While he kept the treadmill at the same speed for each participant, he gradually increased the incline of the running surface, instructing individuals to stop once they felt exhausted. He correlated the results of that long-time experiment with VO2 max, and then organized the data into categories with male and female age percentiles. To this day, the Cooper Institute's numbers are the gold standard for physical assessments, used by law enforcement and many other industries.

I should also say that Dr. Cooper lives what he preaches. He turned ninety in March 2021 and has logged more than eighty thousand miles while exercising daily, whether running (in his younger days) or now walking and cycling.[11]

HEALTHIER US INITIATIVE

In the months that followed the 9/11 attacks, President Bush wanted to shift the nation's attention from death to health. That summer he launched the "HealthierUS Initiative," encouraging and equipping Americans to live longer, better, and healthier lives. He and his advisors had designed the initiative to help Americans of all ages improve their personal health and fitness. The initiative had four main facets:

- Help Americans to be physically active every day
- Help Americans to eat a nutritious diet
- Encourage Americans to get preventive health screenings
- Help Americans to make healthier choices

We know that many chronic diseases can be prevented with modest exercise. In many cases, simple walking for at least a half an hour every day does wonders. Many other physical activities also provide significant benefits. Getting outdoors with children, friends, and family is highly beneficial. The "Be Physically Active Every Day" part of the initiative offered weekends in national parks at no cost. A special website promoted the use of public lands and waters and highlighted conservation assistance with rivers and trails.

Under the heading "Eat a Nutritious Diet," the president suggested that if Americans were to make simple adjustments to their diet—basically portion control and increasing the amount of fruit and vegetables they ate—they could lower their risk of getting cancer and suffering strokes, heart disease, and osteoporosis. The administration enhanced the "Five a Day for Better Health" nutrition curriculum and education in the schools, as well as created the "Eat Smart, Play Hard" campaign.

As a physician who focuses on primary care and prevention, I felt most excited about the initiative's support for Americans to get preventive screenings. Simple things like a cholesterol screen, a blood pressure check, and healthy changes in diet and behavior all are important. The "Healthy Communities Innovation" initiative increased efforts to raise awareness of diabetes screening and improved preventive screenings covered through Medicare.

We've learned from social determinants of health that one of the largest contributors to better health is making healthier choices. Therefore, messages about avoiding tobacco, illicit drugs, and abuse of alcohol were all part of the drug-free communities program. Wise bicycle use and safety also were encouraged.

Many of President Bush's initiatives were based in some way on the work of Dr. Ken Cooper, who talked a great deal about how twenty-first-century medicine emphasized preventive medicine and health promotion. What was true back then is still true today. Most Americans can live longer and better lives if they eliminate cigarette use, reduce inactivity, and decrease obesity. Dr. Cooper's landmark studies also documented the effects of cardiovascular fitness on decreasing the public's utilization of healthcare resources, resulting in substantial national savings.

HEALTH FAIR ON THE EIGHTEEN ACRES

During the first week of summer in 2002, the WHMU provided a health fair for anyone who worked on the Eighteen Acres. That Monday, we offered blood pressure evaluation and weight assessment. We also had cholesterol and glucose testing, with blood tests supported by the air force staff at Malcolm Grow Medical Center. In addition, we did body fat measurements, working in conjunction with the White House Athletic Center staff.

On Tuesday, we offered food for a scheduled three-mile race, with FDA clinical nutritionist Lieutenant Kristen Moe in attendance. At the same time, we offered a presentation on exercise prescription, presented by a physical therapist from the army, Captain Patty Ireland.

On Wednesday, another physical therapist, Rachel Miller, did running evaluations on a treadmill of anyone who requested it. We also had a clinical sports psychologist from the navy, Dr. Andy Davidson, who worked with individuals to mentally prepare for the three-miler scheduled for later. Chaplain Bob Williams, the chaplain both at HMX-1 and then later at Camp David, gave a presentation called "Running the Race of Life."

On Thursday, we participated in a Presidential Health Fair on the South Lawn that dovetailed with President Bush's HealthierUS Initiative. On Friday, we offered summer solstice skin exams by the expert dermatologist from Walter Reed, Dr. Rick Keller. And on Saturday, June 22, President Bush led the White House staff and others in running the Presidential Three-Miler.

Three days after that, we offered a kind of tongue-in-cheek injury assessment for those who ran the three-miler, offered by an orthopedic surgeon from Walter Reed, Dr. Kevin Murphy. Finally, Captain Patty Ireland gave a talk about preparing for the next run.

The WHMU coordinated all these events—not as policy, not as politics, but to provide trusted medical advice and to support the work of the president in urging all Americans to live a better life through fitness.

7

PRESIDENTIAL TRAVEL

The White House makes hundreds of trips a year to scores of domestic and overseas locations. The job of the White House Medical Unit is to prepare and provide medical care at these destinations, thus making sure that the president and other protectees can remain at top performance as they do the important work of the American people.

AROUND THE WORLD

My presidential travel began with President Clinton. During his second term in office, the president visited Africa, India, South America, Asia, the Middle East, New Zealand, and Canada. As the Marine One flight surgeon, I deployed on overseas trips supporting the HMX-1 squadron as they supported the president's travel. The flight surgeon provides care to the deployed marines assigned for that trip, whether abroad or in garrison. Deployments in the continental US have good healthcare resources available to them, so the flight surgeon normally was assigned to support only foreign destinations on overseas swings.

Those trips with President Clinton gave me many great travel experiences and afforded me lots of learning opportunities. I gained expertise in how to assess medical capabilities in other countries, especially as they pertain to the president and those who travel with him.

In March 1998, President Clinton embarked on an eleven-day, six-country tour across the vast continent of Africa, with stops in Ghana, Uganda (where he met with five Central African presidents), Rwanda, and South Africa. Flying home westward, he had official stops in Botswana and Senegal.

When I recall the most memorable trips I took with President Clinton, I think of this trip to Cape Town, South Africa—my very first time covering a presidential visit. The trip to Cape Town also represented my first time on the African continent.

Cape Town, a gorgeous city overflowing with natural beauty, is also full of remarkable history. Table Mountain rises above the city, while Table Bay, with the Indian Ocean to the east and the Atlantic Ocean to the west, frames it. The city has extensive picturesque vineyards, wonderful food, gorgeous temperatures, and breathtaking scenery.

President Clinton's schedule called for him to address parliament. I couldn't help but stare at the parliamentary buildings, both old and new. An older one, reminiscent of a British legislative hall, harkened back to colonial days. In that building, a prime minister had been mortally wounded. Close by stood a new, colorful structure, built by the Nelson Mandela–led African National Congress, which lent a much more modern look to democracy in the twenty-first century. On this memorable trip, we could see for ourselves the long history of the nation's difficult struggle for democracy through the centuries.

On game day, just before the scheduled administrative lift, I was pre-positioned on Robben Island near the landing zone. During a rehearsal, the helo's rotors had kicked up debris, rocks, and other small projectiles from that site, so it was decided I should be ready at that spot in case some bit of flying flotsam or jetsam injured someone who then might need medical treatment. I was therefore waiting on Robben Island near the helicopter landing zone when President and Mrs. Clinton flew in on Marine One.

My unique perch also gave me a wonderful vantage point from which to see the South African Air Force fly in, with its distinctive red helicopters, and land in the proper protocol order at the designated spot. We had scheduled some rehearsal lifts in conjunction with the South African Air Force, so we knew ahead of time how the event would play out.

I watched as President Nelson Mandela and Winnie Mandela got off their aircraft. I believe they were separated at the time, but they still had a unique relationship. The pair warmly greeted President and Mrs. Clinton, and, in that moment, I felt privileged to watch history unfold.

I observed the Clintons and the Mandelas walk arm-in-arm to a minibus that took them past the rock quarry where Madiba (a family or clan name for President Mandela, used as a sign of respect and affection) had worked for seventeen years at hard labor, his sentence for activities that some would characterize as terrorist acts. The two couples later visited the prison where Mr. Mandela had languished for so long. I envisioned him looking out past his barred window, across Table Bay, and watching as the modern city of Cape Town rose into the sky.

In his memoirs, President Mandela wrote that he could have been a better husband. He could have been a better father. But when he was released from prison in 1990 and became the leader of the Republic of South Africa and the father of a reborn nation, he purposefully put retribution and revenge aside and chose reconciliation instead. I believe that's what made him a great leader. His choice proved to be a remarkable one for South Africa's transition from apartheid to a post-apartheid democracy, the best choice for his country and for the world. I hope that this crucial lesson continues to resonate through the ages.

Three months later, in June, President Clinton did a ten-day, five-city swing through China. In 1998, Beijing still teemed with bicycles and had not yet fully transitioned to the modern city that it is today.

In addition to a state visit, President Clinton made a trek to the Forbidden City and to the Great Wall of China. I especially recall his visit to Guilin, where he took a boat ride down the Li River. Our helicopters provided standby support for that visit. Arguably more spectacular than cruising down the river was sitting in the cabin during our familiarization flight, drinking in the karst landscape of the Guilin basin. With its spectacular topography of ridges, towers, fissures, sinkholes, and similar features produced by a landscape underlain by eroded limestone, artists have found it an inspiration for millennia. I love EPCOT at Walt Disney World in Orlando, Florida, and its "Reflections of China" film is my favorite, but the real-life experience is far better!

It's always unique working with the Chinese military and its approach to operations—lots of rules without apparent reason. A Chinese military member was present as an observer on our familiarization flight, but he slept the entire time, so I'm not sure what he observed.

TRAVEL TEAMS

Whether traveling at home or abroad, a multifaceted team always provides continuity for the office of the president. A White House physician and a critical care nurse travel with the team, along with a tactical medical officer, who can be a qualified physician or physician assistant (PA) who has experience in trauma stabilization, advanced airway management, and casualty management of the CBRNE (chemical, biological, radiological, or nuclear event) response.

Providing care anywhere means being prepared to meet the unique threats posed by travel to various locations around the world. Our unique training for care anywhere included a global medicine course, deployment experience, joint planning, orientation and training for advances (both inside and outside the continental US), and protocol/diplomacy training. Speaking additional languages was always helpful.

When we had a protectee actively snow skiing or horse riding, we made sure that assigned team members were current on the activity and familiar with wilderness medicine concepts.

"Care at home" didn't refer only to the Eighteen Acres of the White House grounds, but also to the Naval Observatory, the home of the vice president. President Bush had a second home at the Prairie Chapel Ranch in Texas. President Obama's second residence was on the south side of Chicago near Chicago Fire Department Engine 60. Camp David often serves as the designated retreat.

Sometimes, the vice president would spend time at his second residence as well. For Dick Cheney, that meant Jackson Hole, Wyoming. Joe Biden had residences in Delaware and frequently vacationed in the Caribbean.

Presidential healthcare while away from Washington, D.C., has always been complex, but it has become even more so in recent decades because of increasingly frequent trips to a wide variety of destinations. In 2010, for example, President Obama visited 104 US cities and fourteen foreign countries. That same year, Vice President Joe Biden made 161 domestic stops and visited seventeen foreign countries, while the First Lady, Michelle Obama, visited fifty-seven cities. For the 2010 calendar year, the WHMU supported a total of 567 such trips; in 2011, the number was 548. An average week had more than ten trips for the unit to cover.

I've visited about ninety countries to evaluate their healthcare resources, either for the president or for those providing care for the traveling presidential party. During pre-advance trips, we would assess the local resources, especially the medical resources available to the president and the traveling White House party. In conjunction with the Secret Service, the WHMU would set up a designated hospital, as well as any alternate hospitals. All of this was recorded in a database as a resource for later visits to the same location.

We used Shoreland's cutting-edge, state-of-the-art travel recommendations issued by Travax through an agreement with the Department of Defense. It listed all our planned locations, the capabilities there, and the region's specific threats to health.

We met with local EMS teams to acquire relevant names and contact information, and to understand the local, regional, and state resources. The Secret Service worked with local EMS teams to secure the services of a local ambulance to travel with the presidential motorcade. We did all of this so we could continually be ready to deliver superior protective medicine.

A SHORT HISTORY OF CAMP DAVID

Everybody needs a break from the grind, including presidents. While most US presidents spend most of their time at the White House and in and around Washington D.C., the presidential retreat known as Camp David provides both a place to relax and unwind—an important part of presidential care—as well as an alternate, less formal location for important meetings with leaders from around the world.

The history of Camp David goes back to the early, dark days of World War II after the attack on Pearl Harbor and America's entry into the war. It has been designed as a place of privacy and relaxation for the president and the First Family, a spot where the mind, body, and spirit can be rejuvenated.

President Franklin D. Roosevelt's staff wanted a place suitable for the president's use as a retreat. His personal physician, Ross McIntyre, recommended a location with some elevation and cool temperatures to get him out of the swamp that is D.C. during the summer. At the same time, it needed to be relatively close to the nation's capital. But above all, it had to be a place where security could be maintained.

In the 1930s, the Department of the Interior built several camps employing workers hired by the Depression-era Works Progress Administration and Civilian Conservation Corps. Laborers used local timber, including chestnut and oak trees, to build these facilities. They built some cabins in the Catoctin Mountains on the border of Maryland and Pennsylvania. President Roosevelt selected one of those camps in 1942 to become his retreat. We always knew this as "camp number three," but the presidential retreat was officially known as Camp Hi-Catoctin.

President Roosevelt used the code name "Shangri-La" to refer to the presidential retreat during the last few years of his life. He used it to hold conferences with his military advisors and to get away and recuperate from Washington, D.C. He also had one secret visit there with Britain's prime minister, Winston Churchill, to discuss Allied war efforts.

President Truman, the next commander in chief, did not use the presidential retreat as frequently as FDR did. He did, however, decide to keep it open year-round instead of being only a summertime retreat. That meant the buildings had to be modified to include steam heat to make them bearable during the winter months, especially at the high elevation. He also made the retreat open to members of his staff, and not only when he and Mrs. Truman were present. Somebody on President Truman's staff used Shangri-La nearly every week during his administration.

A seismic political change occurred in 1953 with the election of Republican Dwight D. Eisenhower as president. Name changes often follow a new party in power. President Eisenhower renamed the retreat Camp David after his grandson, David Eisenhower. The president used it as a place to relax, but he also held some important events there, including hosting Soviet premier Nikita Khrushchev. During that time, when the United States began employing a more friendly approach toward world problems, the phrase "the spirit of Camp David" was coined—by Krushchev, of all people. (The peaceful rhetoric didn't keep his forces from shooting down an American U-2 spy plane in May 1960, however.)

After President Eisenhower's eight years in office, President Kennedy took over as commander in chief in 1961. Although he was a Democrat, he chose to stick with the name Camp David, and the designation has remained to this day. President Kennedy and his young family used many of the facilities on the presidential retreat and often walked around the grounds, enjoying nature. Camp David also was a favorite place for Mrs. Kennedy and her two young children during the thousand days of Camelot. They often rode horses there.

President Lyndon B. Johnson used Camp David for conferences and meetings with foreign leaders. Primarily, however, he used it as a getaway from the hustle and bustle of D.C.

President Richard Nixon and his family also used Camp David to relax, and there he also hosted Leonid Brezhnev, the new Soviet premier. Eleven times he invited other foreign leaders to meet there during his time in office.

President Ford used Camp David infrequently, visiting only occasionally. In July 1975, he met there with President Suharto of Indonesia.

President Jimmy Carter and his family, along with members of his administration, used Camp David extensively during his four years in office. President Carter met with President Anwar Sadat of Egypt at Camp David in February 1978. Later that year, in September, President Carter, President Sadat, and Prime Minister Menachem Begin of Israel met for thirteen days at Camp David, conducting Middle East peace negotiations. History remembers their accomplishments as the Camp David Accords. They met in a cabin then called Laurel, today known as Holly. To this day, I remember using the tables in that cabin and seeing the documents from the 1978 peace accords.

President Reagan may have the record for the most days spent at Camp David. He made sure that every day he was there he would walk and swim and take horseback rides along the extensive nature trails built for his use. During his time in office, President Reagan had a breakfast meeting with President José López Portillo of Mexico (June 1981), hosted Margaret Thatcher, the British prime minister (December 1984 and November 1986), and spent a day with Yasuhiro Nakasone, Japan's prime minister (April 1986), all at Camp David. He also held several meetings with members of Congress, his cabinet, and other administration officials. Many of President Reagan's weekly radio broadcasts originated from Camp David. He would typically walk over to Laurel Cabin to do the weekly broadcast, and then head outside, get on his horse, and enjoy nature.

A couple of decades later, workers converted these horseback trails into mountain biking trails for President George W. Bush. If he was at Camp David when his weekly radio broadcast had to be done, he

JEFFREY KUHLMAN, MD, MPH

tended to follow the pattern of President Reagan. After finishing the broadcast, he'd leave the cabin and go running or bike riding.

President George H. W. Bush was very familiar with Camp David because he had served for eight years as vice president under President Reagan. Both he and First Lady Barbara Bush spent a lot of time at Camp David. During his four years in office, Bush 41 used Camp David extensively as a place of business gatherings, entertaining, and relaxation. He invited many foreign leaders to Camp David, including the president of Mexico; the prime minister of Australia; the West German chancellor; Margaret Thatcher and John Major, prime ministers of the United Kingdom; the king and queen of Spain; the president of Turkey; the Soviet premier Mikhail Gorbachev; President Boris Yeltsin of Russia; and the first president of Ukraine, Leonid Kravchuk.

Possibly more than any other First Family, the Bushes actively engaged in the recreational endeavors available at Camp David, including jogging, playing tennis, horseshoes, golf, volleyball, bike riding, and skeet shooting. The grounds also boast a movie theater, game room, pool table, bowling alley, and library. Every day, Bush 41 would take a brisk, long walk along the nature trails or around the compound's perimeter.

Two decades later, when the former president visited Camp David as a guest of his son, Bush 43, he would come down on the weekend and play wallyball with me and the military staff.

In 1993, Bill Clinton became president. In his first year, he tended to use Camp David as a weekend retreat for his management team. In his second year, he started using it more frequently. He and the First Family actively participated in church services at Evergreen Chapel, where on occasion he was known to sing as a member of the choir.

President George W. Bush was very familiar with Camp David from his previous visits as a family member during the administrations of both President Reagan and his father, Bush 41. It seemed to me that the president enjoyed the nature of Camp David much more than he did city life at 1600 Pennsylvania Avenue. Every day, he would either run three miles or mountain bike for an hour. He also frequently used the Camp David fitness center, known as Wye Oak. He figured out ways to hit golf balls and skeet shoot, and he and his family used Camp David for informal get-togethers, extended family reunions, and holiday family time.

During an early 2007 visit, Bush 43 invited me and the camp nurse to watch a movie in the Camp David theater—a first invitation for me. We enjoyed *The Last King of Scotland*, a historical drama about a young Scottish doctor who intersected with and cared for the Ugandan dictator and president, Idi Amin. At times entertaining and at times brutal, the film provided me with both a memorable experience and an unusual setting.

President Obama probably held the largest international meeting at Camp David when he invited the leaders of the G8 nations to a summit there in 2012.

Today, about a dozen cabins exist on the premises. The largest, Laurel Lodge, has three conference rooms, a dining room, and a small presidential office. Hickory Lodge hosts indoor recreational activities and offers a grill, bar, and gift shop, as well as the theater. Holly Cabin has smaller meeting rooms and some recreational space.

Eight decades after Camp David was built, the cabins still look very rustic with their board and batten construction, all painted moss green. Appropriately enough, the landscape is all native vegetation, perfect for a little rest and relaxation—just what the doctor ordered.

HEALTHCARE AT CAMP DAVID

I was the first White House physician assigned to serve as the Camp David physician, remaining in that capacity from 2003 to 2005. Previously, a navy physician assigned to Bethesda had provided administrative oversight.

During that time, I also completed a master of public health (MPH) at Johns Hopkins, in addition to a postdoctoral fellowship in occupational and environmental medicine. I maintained my top-secret security clearance and discovered that while the commute to Baltimore was a few more miles than the commute to the White House, it took less time. Subsequently, I passed boards in occupational medicine and became board certified in aerospace medicine.

My Camp David duties included monthly visits to the retreat site, organizing and overseeing its medical care and capabilities, and making sure that any existing or new contingency areas could adequately provide medical care. The medical capabilities of Camp David include a cabin named Eucalyptus, used for anyone stationed there or who comes as a guest. During non-presidential visit times, a navy independent duty corpsman staffs it, while during a presidential visit, it's supplemented by the White House physician and a White House nurse, who remain on duty for the entire presidential visit.

We had a unique situation where some older buildings developed indoor air quality concerns. I utilized my new occupational medicine training to expeditiously address those problems. We certainly didn't want guests or valued team members getting sick or dying on the grounds! To my knowledge, no one has ever died at Camp David.

PRESIDENTIAL MOTORCADES

Presidential motorcades carry their own risks. In November 2006, I rode in a motorcade with President Bush during a visit to Honolulu as we returned from the annual Asia-Pacific Economic Cooperation (APEC) Summit. We drove through Hickam Air Force Base at a slow speed. A Honolulu motorcycle police officer raced past us and suffered a collision ahead of us on the base and died of his injuries five days later.

Within a year—on August 27, 2007—as we headed to the Albuquerque airport, a police officer on a motorcycle suffered a major accident. His back wheel slid out and hit a curb, and he was thrown twenty feet through the air, slamming into a tree. I released the local EMS ambulance to assist him and dispatched the White House medical advance officer, a physician assistant. Unfortunately, the police officer died at the trauma center at the University of New Mexico Hospital.

During the Obama administration, while traveling in Jupiter, Florida, I witnessed a bad motorcycle accident in which an officer went down on the interstate while protecting an entrance ramp. A driver watching the motorcade didn't see the officer and plowed into him.

Local EMS officials must understand that the primary function of the ambulance in a presidential detail is to treat and transport the president. But they also need to consider having a contingency plan to assist a downed officer (or similar personnel) when appropriate or as directed by the Secret Service. No official records are kept of such accidents, but unofficial records say about one incident like those occurs every other year.

PRESIDENTIAL TRAVEL WITH OBAMA

A new president's first foreign trip is traditionally made to our neighbors to the north, Canada. So, on February 19, 2009, I accompanied President Obama to Ottawa, the country's capital. I remember the grandeur of the Gothic Revival buildings we briefly visited and how our motorcade made an unscheduled stop for the president to greet cheering onlookers. Reggie Love, my backseat companion in the spare limo, served as the president's "body man," his personal assistant. Reggie brought a pastry called a beaver tail into the limo and we had our first taste of the fried dough treat. Good thing I carried hand sanitizer in my medical supplies.

The first truly overseas swing came at the end of March and into the first week of April. It was a nine-day, six-country trip. We stopped first in London at the G20 Summit, where President Obama met with the prime minister of the United Kingdom as well as with the leader of the opposition. He also met with Queen Elizabeth II and a few royal family members. The queen and Prince Philip gave the president a signed, official photo of themselves, along with an invitation to come back and stay at Buckingham Palace when his schedule allowed.

I thought, *What do you give a queen who has everything she desires? Maybe a set of CDs with her favorite show tunes?*

For our second stop, we headed to Strasbourg, France, and Baden-Baden, Germany, as the two countries jointly hosted the NATO Summit. Next up was the US-EU Summit in Prague. On the way home, we had an overnight visit to Turkey's capital city, Ankara, with a final stop in Baghdad en route home. President Obama was all business on this trip, actively engaged in all the summits and meeting the other world leaders for the first time. He was the new kid on the block but very much the center of attention, with many testing his leadership abilities on a new stage. He rose to the challenge. The First Lady accompanied him on part of the schedule, but since the school year was still in session, their daughters couldn't travel with them.

FOREIGN TRAVEL

Anywhere the president goes in the world, a White Top helicopter waits to provide any medical response required. The president and his staff log hundreds of hours a year on Air Force One, a Boeing 747-200 with a fully equipped medical compartment. Its onboard medical limitations are related more to the expertise and skills of the physician and nurse onboard than to the equipment or the supplies available on the plane.

Travel to foreign countries can involve many personal injury threats, whether related to modes of transportation, walking, motorcades, cycles, or other causes. We also labored to remain aware of good, old-fashioned safety and security concerns regarding risky areas to be visited.

We had to consider the complex, chronic medical conditions that can arise in medically resource–challenged locations. Updated health and safety information had to be vetted, making sure it correctly outlined the relevant health threats. At the same time, it had to address the safety and security of the planned transport modes, the lodging, and the various venues we planned to visit. We made sure that personal meds were readily available, whether for pre-existing conditions, acute conditions that might pop up, or prophylaxis, as appropriate.

We took appropriate precautions against insect-borne illnesses, as many travel threats come from insects—not only malaria, but also dengue fever, chikungunya, and tick-borne illnesses. We had to know how to respond to such threats, as well as to dog bites, monkey bites, and snake bites. Any of these could end somebody's trip, seriously impact their effectiveness, or cause permanent disability or even death. We also routinely prepared for common food and water-borne illnesses, such as traveler's diarrhea.

Continuity planning included ensuring that travel insurance was active, whether local medical support was available, and whether individuals needed access to their personal health and allergy records to receive basic medical services or first aid. Many countries require immunizations, such as for yellow fever, which means documentation for such vaccinations must be readily available.

As the physician to the president, I remained active with the International Society of Travel Medicine and demonstrated expertise with my certification of traveler health (CTH). In August 2011, in Lima, Peru, I also completed a multi-week Gorgas course in advanced tropical medicine available to infectious disease experts. I learned about a variety of tropical diseases and saw firsthand how to diagnose and treat such cases.

Prior to 2014, global mortality stats focused on infectious disease as the leading cause of death. But after 2014, for the first time in world history, deaths from noncommunicable diseases surpassed deaths from infectious diseases. A standard focus on vaccine-preventable illnesses, vector-borne diseases, and public health challenges such as food and water are just the tip of the iceberg.

Knowing *all* of that was not just a "nice to have" but was also an imperative of the job.

A MEMORABLE FINAL TRIP

My last trip supporting President Obama took place in July 2013, accompanied by the First Lady and his two daughters. The very last stop of our trip occurred in Cape Town, where I had visited the first time with President Clinton nearly sixteen years before, back in January 1998. President Mandela's heart was still beating and he lived in Johannesburg at the time of President Obama's trip, but his body and mind could not handle a visit. Unfortunately, he died just a few weeks later.

With President Obama, I found myself back on Robben Island. There I saw the president gain a better understanding of the gravity and the symbolism of Nelson Mandela, along with the undertones of both world leadership and race. I also saw the traits that had made both presidents Nobel Peace Prize laureates.

I consider my two trips to South Africa amazing bookends for the sixteen privileged years I supported presidential travel. When others hear about my medical career, they often ask, "What is the best thing about working at the White House?" I know I should say "the people," but often I say "the travel."

"Okay," they reply, "then what's the worst thing about working at the White House?"

"The travel," I tell them.

Twenty twelve was an election year for President Obama. He took about two hundred trips that year in which he left Washington, D.C., used Air Force One, and went on business travel for his job. Of those two hundred, we made sure that a White House physician and a White House nurse were always on board to provide medical care to the president, for anyone traveling with him, and for anyone connected to the president who might need medical care. In that year of the two hundred trips, I accompanied the president about 120 times.

Others often ask me with genuine curiosity, "Did you ever see Air Force One?"

"Well, yes," I explain, "that's how we got around."

I went on hundreds of trips but unfortunately never got any frequent flyer miles, although I was able to log flight time for my navy flight pay. I also developed good personal and professional relationships with the flight attendants and pilots who provided the president with unparalleled service. They are true heroes of presidential support.

When the time comes for a trip, if it's good weather, the president typically walks out from the Oval Office, strides across the South Lawn, and gets on the waiting White Top helicopter by climbing the front stairway to the aircraft after saluting the marines. His traveling staff, military aide, and physician get on last, just before the Secret Service detail. The helo takes them to Joint Base Andrews, where they board Air Force 1.

In more than a decade of White House service, I was privileged to take hundreds of trips on Marine One. How many? I can't say for sure. The only thing I know for certain is that the marines don't give frequent flyer miles, either. But the other rewards are priceless and helped me be in the right place to render care.

8

CARE UNDER FIRE
AND BEING READY

Medical training for traumas in the late twentieth century basical-ly gave the following advice: give the victim lots of fluids, pro-tect the cervical spine, and get them to a hospital via an ambulance. In the early 2000s, with the development of protective medicine—a well-equipped, well-trained healthcare professional embedded with a protective detail—the optimal care under fire for penetrating trauma, knife attack, or gunshot wound dramatically changed. Physicians were instructed to pay attention to vital signs and the shock index (pulse divided by systolic blood pressure); carry and use prehospital whole blood; carry TXA (tranexamic acid) and give a bolus early, keeping the blood in the body; and get to definitive care (a Level I trauma center) as soon as possible by the most rapid means. Intravenous fluids and cervical collars were no longer necessary. The "golden hour of trau-ma" is made up and too long. The lessons from battlefield medicine, learned in Afghanistan and Iraq, were embraced by the WHMU. Two decades later, medical training is slow to adopt these lessons, and aca-demics still debate their effectiveness.

IN THE LINE OF FIRE

Unfortunately, as we've seen, presidents are in the line of fire, whether at home or abroad. Four US presidents have died at the hands of assassins, and many more have survived assassination attempts. In all four of the assassinations, gunshot wounds were the cause of death, whether directly or through later complications.

Like most things in medicine, prevention is always the best treatment, and we rely upon the expertise of the United States Secret Service to keep our leaders safe. They think about prevention nonstop. But despite their hard work and many precautions taken, sometimes it isn't enough.

When someone is shot, death happens within seconds about 25 percent of the time. If a bullet hits the heart, the great vessels, or a substantial part of the head, the victim will die almost immediately, regardless of the time and location of any definitive care provided. The only way to improve those odds is to work to make sure the individual doesn't get hit, or to provide the person with improved body armor or better defensive tactics. In combat, the immediate death rate from gunfire has been reduced from 25 percent to 20 percent.

Individuals who survive "instant death" make it to something called "the golden hour." The largest percentage of gunshot victims who die within that hour—10 percent—perish from exsanguination (they bleed out) or from complications obstructing the airway. To prevent that, doctors work hard to keep the blood in the body and make sure that the airway stays open.

During the first six hours, another 10 percent die from complications associated with breathing problems (technically speaking, either through ventilatory-perfusion mismatch, tension pneumothorax, cardiac tamponade, or other injuries that cause significant breathing problems). If the victims survive those six hours, the primary cause of death in the first twenty-four hours is shock, usually from hemorrhagic shock. Among those who survive the first twenty-four hours and yet die, death often occurs from an infection leading to sepsis (if this takes place more than seventy-two hours after the gunshot wound).

We've seen these conditions play out in American presidential history. Military medicine speaks of this phenomenon as "the die-off curve": instant death, the golden hour, the first six hours, six to twenty-four hours, and the seventy-two-plus hours. *Military Medicine* published this progression in 1996 in reference to tactical combat.[12] I read these articles, embraced them, discussed the material with their authors, took hands-on field courses at the FBI Academy and Mayo Clinic in Scottsdale, and then implemented them as our standard operating procedure at the WHMU.

CARE UNDER FIRE

What we call "care under fire" has four unique phases.

Phase One: Prevent the Individual from Getting Hit Again

If the protectee gets hit, we take action to try to prevent the individual from getting hit again. If he's able to speak, then the airway is okay. In blunt trauma, we spend extraordinary amounts of time protecting the cervical spine—we put on a neck brace or use a full body board. But in penetrating trauma, when bullets fly and one hits the cervical spine, there's not much we can do to prevent further injury. If it's not indicated to immobilize the cervical spine, it's not necessary to do anything else for it.

Phase Two: Keep the Blood in the Body

In the first few minutes, we aim to establish an airway and stop any life-threatening hemorrhaging. An oral or nasopharyngeal airway is simple and effective. If a patient is unconscious, inserting a laryngeal mask airway (LMA) works in the field, even if the care provider can't clearly see what he or she is doing. Keeping the blood in the body may involve using bandages, direct pressure, and tourniquets. Antifibrinolytics or hemostatic treatments can be used, along with other measures, to keep the blood in the body.

Phase Three: Perform Tactical Field Care

Within the first hour, we treat complications employing tactical field care. We decompress the chest, if necessary. We were taught, "If you do only two things—put a tourniquet on and relieve a tension pneumothorax—then you can probably avoid 70–90 percent of all preventable deaths on the battlefield." We consider using chest tubes and intravenous fluids, administer oxygen, and continue to manage the airway.

Phase Four: Get the Patient to Definitive Care

Definitive care usually means a hospital with an operating room and an experienced surgical team standing by. While no official national trauma network of hospitals in the US exists, each state has its own trauma designation and program offering various levels of complexity. There also should be additional medical equipment on board the casualty evacuation vehicle (ambulance, truck, helicopter, etc.)

When medical personnel have trained for and implemented this kind of combat casualty care, and the injured party receives advanced life support for no longer than the first six hours until getting to surgical care, the mortality rate drops to about 1 percent. We saw this play out during the Gulf War (0.4 percent), Desert Storm, Desert Shield, and in Bosnia (1.8 percent).

ACS Capital Plan

After President Reagan was shot in 1981, the American College of Surgeons Committee on Trauma developed something called the Capital Program. It identifies verified trauma centers, not only in the US but also around the world. Before then, protective details would often roll into town and hear local law enforcement personnel make comments like, "The hospital we want to use is the one where my grandmother got taken care of after she fell and broke her hip. They gave her really good care."

While that's nice, it may not be the best choice for acute trauma. Often you may need to go to the hospital in a not-so-nice part of town, sometimes known as the "knife and gun club." Why? They have the necessary experience and are always ready. And that's where the best definitive care is.

There are two general types of traumas: penetrating trauma from bullets and knives, and blunt trauma from incidents such as falls or car accidents. Those are two *very* different types of trauma. For care under fire, you want the most experienced, capable, trained people possible who take care of penetrating types of injuries every day.

The gold standard for definitive care is a Level I trauma center verified with the Capital Plan. There are also Level II, Level III, and unrated trauma centers. Verified trauma centers list the regional trauma surgeon, the trauma medical director, and the trauma program manager. The WHMU still uses the Capital Program for White House travel.

Trained to Deliver Care Under Fire

At the WHMU, we established a training protocol unique to care under fire. We made sure everyone on the unit got operational emergency medical skills training (OEMS), also known as field medic training. Some went through SWAT team medic training.

The military offered a course on the medical management of chemical and biological casualties that also covered the medical effects of ionizing radiation, basic and advanced cardiac life support, and advanced trauma life support. All nurses completed either the trauma nursing core course or the advanced trauma care for nurses (TNCC or ATNC). We also made sure that everybody did a trauma rotation at a trauma center.

For care in the air, we had to be able to quickly transport critically ill patients to a designated medical treatment facility. Humans encounter unique medical problems once they escape the Earth's surface and rise into a high-altitude, low-pressure environment. Whether a helicopter carries the president as Marine One, or a fixed-wing aircraft carries the president as Air Force One, we must provide care with qualified personnel and equipment. Some of us had flight nurse or flight surgeon designations, and many had critical care air transport (CCAT) training. To complete our flight physiology training, everyone in the WHMU had to pass ingress and egress training for both fixed-wing and rotary-wing aircraft.

As the associate director for plans and training, I wrote a training mission statement for the White House Medical Unit: "We care . . . under fire, in the air, in crisis, at home, and anywhere."

For those who say, "It will never happen here," I would point to history. We've suffered at least three major tragedies in NASA alone. On January 27, 1967, *Apollo 1* lost astronauts Virgil Grissom, Edward White, and Roger Chafee during routine ground testing of their *Apollo* capsule when fire engulfed their pure oxygen, highly compressed air environment.

As a medical student at Loma Linda, I observed the launch of the space shuttle *Challenger* on January 28, 1986. Just seventy-three seconds after takeoff, I watched in horror as the shuttle erupted in a fireball, killing the entire seven-member crew.

During President Bush's first term, on February 1, 2003, I watched on television as the space shuttle *Columbia* broke apart upon re-entry at the end of a sixteen-day scientific mission, killing an entire crew for a second time.

That one struck a bit closer to home, as crew members David Brown and Laura Clark were both members of the navy flight surgeon community and were friends of friends. The tragedy happened while I was covering a presidential trip. I returned home the next day and went to work at the White House, when it was announced that the president would visit Johnson Space Center in Houston to pay his respects. The physician to the president, Dr. Tubb, himself a NASA finalist (ironically with Drs. Brown and Clark), asked me to do the advance for that trip.

I immediately got up from our breakfast at the White House mess, walked out of the Executive Mansion, boarded the metro heading to

Ronald Reagan Washington National Airport, and hopped on the next nonstop flight to Houston, where I joined the White House advance preparations team. We updated our advance planning by getting the appropriate trauma hospitals in place. Only then did I call home to let my supportive wife know what had happened. I bought a toothbrush, along with other essentials for the presidential visit the next day, and returned home on Air Force One.

Care in crisis includes critical incident stress management, continuity of the presidency training, and assault on the principal (AOP) exercises. We also visited the contingency hospital sites to verify their capabilities and to ensure they were prepared.

We continually checked to make sure everyone stayed up to date on primary medical care, acute medical care, emergency medical care, disaster preparedness and response, complementary alternative medicine, prevention of disease and wellness, and coordination of specialty care. We made mental wellness available for all those on the Eighteen Acres who supported the president in some capacity. We also ensured that they had access to evaluation, crisis intervention services, and spiritual readiness tools for family and personal counseling as well as critical incidents.

Finally, we worked hard to ensure that all medical providers stayed current in their state medical licensure, continuing medical education, board certification, and specialty-specific training.

READY ON THE FIRST DAY

Basic orientation for the WHMU went something like this: "What do you need to be ready on your first day? What do you need to be ready in your first year? What do you need to be ready for your first duty?"

We started the White House Medical Fellowship for all our newcomers to the unit. The first six months included a clinical rotation, while the next six months focused on operational training. We laid out goals and objectives for the fellowship using a flowchart; phase development and progression; professional competencies; and a list of courses, completions, designations, and presidential service badge certificates, along with appropriate timelines. Presidential or vice presidential duty lasted two years. Some stayed on for an extension and so received appropriate periodic refresher training.

We had a manpower plan tied to a strength and qualification matrix. We maintained training folders. We integrated the scheduling and training qualifications to ensure individuals were ready for their duty assignments.

In 2005, after realizing we had access to many military medical officers who had fresh combat experience from Afghanistan and Iraq, I proposed and initiated a new position to utilize their unique skills. These tactical military officers (TMOs) focus on pre-hospital tactical trauma care and are equipped with a backpack used for both training and practice. They supply the backpack themselves based on a standardized list. They focus on the treatment and management of blunt and penetrating trauma and advanced airway management, whether through a laryngeal mask airway (LMA) or an endotracheal tube with a rapid sequence induction (drugs that paralyze the body to quickly pass a tube through the vocal cords into the trachea). They also focus on hemorrhage control, especially on recognizing and providing initial treatment for injuries caused by chemical and biological sources, along with blast injuries. Most have special training and equipment for extraction, stabilization, packaging up for transport, and casualty evacuation.

Those we recruited to the WHMU needed not only the requisite professional education but also preferred experience in combat emergency medicine, whether pre-hospital or in the traditional emergency department. They also needed experience with special operations and as first responders in the pre-hospital environment. Paramedic EMT training was also helpful, and sometimes they had chem/bio training and experience. We initiated the Presidential Tactical Trauma Training Program (PT-3) based on the philosophy that one must train to be ready for the unexpected day when you need to save a life.

We practiced how we played and played how we practiced.

But more important than all of this was unit fit. Had the recruits been enculturated to show up, do their job, be responsible, be part of a team, and not be an army of one all to themselves? That was especially important because some of our team was integrated with EMT-trained members of the Secret Service as part of a special response unit with the acronym HAMMER (Hazardous Agent Mitigation Medical Emergency Response Team).

PROTECTIVE MEDICINE

Dr. Connie Mariano served as the physician to the president for Bill Clinton from 1993 to 2001. She was a navy medical officer trained in internal medicine, retiring as a rear admiral. Dr. Mariano coined the term "protective medicine."

Over the following decade, I spearheaded an effort to fully develop the concept of protective medicine as the leader of training and operations for the WHMU. We developed its capabilities, trained the people involved, acquired the necessary equipment, and improved the transport protocols.

Protective medicine refers simply to a healthcare professional with the right equipment, training, and experience who is embedded (or "inside the bubble") with a protective detail (that is, men and women carrying weapons as part of their job to protect an individual, known as "the protectee"). The protectee is often a head of state but can be an ultra-high-net-worth individual, such as a celebrity or a rock star.

We've spent a lot of time focusing on trauma care and responding to external threats, but the fact is that the most likely life-threatening event is an out-of-hospital cardiac arrest. In the United States, a thousand individuals every day suffer an out-of-hospital cardiac arrest. Their survival depends largely on how quickly the emergency medical system is activated, how many seconds or minutes elapse until a defibrillator is placed on their chest and activated, and how soon the heart can return to spontaneous circulation.

The out-of-hospital cardiac arrest survival rate in the US hovers in the single-digit percentile. At the WHMU, we tried to improve that rate by making sure that we always had a physician within two minutes of the president—and not just a physician, but one fully trained and experienced with out-of-hospital cardiac arrests, current on training, and skilled with the equipment they carried, including an automated external defibrillator. Regarding the latter, we shifted from the monophasics to the biphasics (the leading edge of the latest technology). We also carried an advanced laryngeal mask airway, an endotracheal tube (size fitting the protectee), and, when appropriate, rapid sequence induction medications.

The gold standard of care is to have a second set of hands during advanced cardiac life support (ACLS), so we also had a critical care nurse present within two minutes. We would carry ACLS medications, along with a portable heart monitor. Another important resource was oxygen, provided by the Secret Service or by local ambulances present at the locations involved or accompanying the motorcade.

The community standard for the time it should take a first responder to employ an automated external defibrillator (AED) in the US is four minutes, and eight minutes for full advanced life support (ALS). For serious trauma, we think of the golden hour and fixed decontamination assets. Then, for patient evacuation, we think of a fixed transport time between two locations.

The WHMU planning cuts all of those in half. Our paradigm was that the first responder employ the AED within two minutes and the full ALS within four minutes. For serious trauma, the first responder was expected to stabilize and reach a Level I ACS trauma center for definitive care in thirty minutes. For chem/bio, they were expected to decontaminate onsite immediately and then cut the patient evacuation time in half by prepositioning transport assets.

Those response times could involve a motorcade; if so, we had fully equipped ambulances, referred to as Medic One. If the travel took place in the D.C. area, we would have access to a Secret Service ambulance called Sunburn, with the George Washington University Hospital just minutes away. At Camp David, we always had HMX that provided either a VH-3 or a VH-60 helicopter, with a short air travel time to a Level I trauma/shock center.

Other important items to have on hand included antihistamines, such as Benadryl or oral-dissolving Claritin, and an antiemetic like Zofran, along with other pain relief medications. We prepared for penetrating trauma, for out-of-hospital cardiac arrests, and for chemical or biological asymmetrical threats (see chapter 9).

To be prepared for the medical effects of the latter, we all completed the necessary training, carried the appropriate personal protective equipment, fit it all into a plan, and then had on hand the appropriate antidotes or medications for the most likely chemical or biological scenarios.

CLINT EASTWOOD'S ADVICE

You can learn a lot about medical care if you watch Clint Eastwood movies. I automatically think of *Dirty Harry*. Consider Harry Callahan's three field medical rules:

- A man's got to know his limitations.
- When you are alone, the sky's the limit.
- Do you feel lucky?

The men and women who care for the president, and for those who support the president, must make sure that they know the relevant field medical rules and that they are fully prepared to provide care everywhere, under all situations, and continually. It also doesn't hurt to remember another Clint Eastwood line: "Being comfortable is overrated."

9

SPECIAL SITUATIONS

In the past, many of us in the United States blithely thought that our vast oceans would provide us with great geographical protection. At first, we believed they would provide us protection against wars; and then later, we thought they would protect us against illnesses and pandemics involving human-to-human transmission.

But oceanic travel and modern warfare made us realize our vulnerability. We saw some of our protection disappear with seafaring wooden ships in the eighteenth and nineteenth centuries, and then more of it vanish with airplanes and missiles in the twentieth century. Today, with commercial air travel making it possible to reach nearly any point on the planet within just a few hours, we understand how little protection those oceans in fact afford us.

During a crisis, whether it be a terrorist attack or the early stages of a pandemic, important communication must take place. The mental imagery we typically have is of someone standing behind a podium placed in front of the US flag in the press room in the West Wing of the White House. At those times, the public wonders two things: *Do they know what they're talking about?* and *Do they care about me?*

Contrasting communication styles exist. Some prefer a forceful and blunt approach like that often used by former president Donald Trump, while others prefer something more akin to the one employed by Anthony Fauci, the former director of the National Institute of Allergy and Infectious Diseases. Regardless of the approach, however, viewers want to feel assured that the speakers know what they're talking about and that they care about the American people.

THE ABCs OF HARMFUL BIOLOGICAL AGENTS

The CDC classifies harmful biological agents into three categories: A, B, and C. The White House Medical Unit must know how to diagnose, prevent, and treat category A biological agents, which can cause high casualties and death. These pathogens disseminate easily and warrant special actions. There are five category A biological agents.

Anthrax occurs naturally in some animal populations and in the soil, causing gastrointestinal symptoms or cutaneous lesions in humans. Anthrax can be weaponized, making the spores airborne and inhaled, causing deadly pulmonary responses.

Tularemia is the second category A biological agent. Also known as rabbit fever, it is caused by the bacterium *Francisella tularensis*. This zoonotic disease is spread to humans either by infected animals (deer flies, rodents, hares, and rabbits) or by contaminated food and water. It causes swelling of the lymph nodes and produces fever, ulcers, rashes, sore throat, vomiting, abdominal pain, and muscle aches.

The third category A agent is *Yersinia pestis*, the causative agent for the disease commonly known as plague. An outbreak in the Middle Ages killed between seventy-five million and two hundred million people, about 30–50 percent of Europe's population. Symptoms include fever, chills, headaches, muscle pain, and swollen lymph glands. A person in Central Oregon made national headlines in February 2024 when it was reported he was diagnosed with plague, contracted through his cat. Both human and feline were treated early on and recovered fully, posing no threat to the community.[13]

The fourth category A agent is *smallpox*, caused by the variola virus. It can spread through the air (sneezing or coughing), through direct contact with body fluids, or through indirect contact (sharing clothing or bedding). It is thought the disease killed three hundred million persons in the twentieth century alone. Symptoms include a rash on the face, hands, forearms, and torso that turns into blisters, along with fever, chills, body aches, malaise, and vomiting.

The fifth category A agents are viruses causing *hemorrhagic fever*. The most well-known fevers are Ebola, Marburg, hantavirus, dengue, Lassa, and yellow fever.

A strategic national stockpile to counter these agents was created a couple of decades ago, originally as a defense for nuclear, biological, and chemical attacks. It contains antibiotics effective against anthrax, tularemia, and plague. Also in the stockpile are vaccines against biological agents, personal protective equipment (disposable gloves and masks), ventilators, auto-injectors for the treatment of chemical agents, and specific medicines for radiological events.

PREPARING FOR BIOLOGICAL AND CHEMICAL THREATS

When a disease event or incident happens, the onset or initial effects of the attack may be insidious. Those effects may be delayed, making it difficult to distinguish bioterrorism from a naturally occurring event. The outbreaks may present similarly.

Preparedness for a pandemic or outbreak—whether man-made or from Mother Nature—and our response to it are intertwined. It's crucial to have both a plan of preparedness and a coordinated response.

I think here of the Tom Clancy novel *Executive Orders*, where the antagonist weaponizes the Ebola virus to make a biological attack on the US. But the greatest natural killer in the history of mankind is the variola virus, the smallpox pathogen. Fortunately, after global vaccination efforts—a modern-day miracle—naturally occurring smallpox was eradicated from the face of the earth in late 1977. There may be two stashes of smallpox left on the planet: one at a special lab at the CDC and another at a lab in Russia.

Our awareness and preparedness for targeted or large-scale biological/chemical threats, whether natural or man-made, have also been transformed since the mid-twentieth century. The White House doctor must know about such threats to the president and to the White House.

During the height of the Cold War, President Nixon made an unexpected trip to Fort Detrick in Frederick, Maryland. On November 25, 1969, he announced the end to all offensive aspects of the US biological weapons program.

A few years later, in 1975, the United States ratified both the 1925 Geneva Protocol on its fiftieth anniversary and the 1972 Biological Weapons Convention; both are international treaties outlawing biological warfare. After 1969, the United States had no offensive biological capability.

And yet, it's critical to retain a strong defense against nuclear, biological, and chemical warfare. For the federal government, that responsibility falls to the Department of Health and Human Services, of which the Centers for Disease Control and Prevention (CDC) is the expert agency.

Around Thanksgiving 2006 a news report about the death of a former Russian spy caught my attention. Alexander Litvinenko, a vocal critic of the Russian government, had died of heart failure. His hair had fallen out, his throat had swollen, and his upper respiratory tract had essentially collapsed. He also had severely compromised immune and neurological systems.

A seriously ill Litvinenko had received treatment at University College Hospital in London, where he died. Officially the death was unexplained, but the deceased's symptoms were consistent with poisoning. As a forty-three-year-old male previously in good health who suddenly became ill with a strange cluster of symptoms, the case raised many questions. His unexplained death could be related to either biological or chemical agents delivered to the former spy by someone who didn't like what he had been saying.

As I write, controversy swirls around yet another death, this time of Alexei Navalny. A Russian dissident and critic of Russian president Vladimir Putin, Navalny had been arrested and sent to an arctic penal colony known as the Polar Wolf prison. The forty-seven-year-old died on February 16, 2024, of causes variously described by Russian sources as "sudden death syndrome," a blood clot, or after taking a brisk walk in the prison. His widow suggested he might have been poisoned with the same nerve agent, Novichok, used on him in August 2020. A human rights group said Navalny had been forced to spend over two and a half hours in an open-air, outdoor solitary confinement space where the temperature can dip to minus 27 degrees Celsius (minus 16.6 degrees Fahrenheit), and afterward received a punch to the heart—a KGB-era method of killing.[14] The United States, in response, announced "substantial" sanctions levied against Russia for the unexplained death (the Russian government had refused to release the body for testing).[15]

REMEMBERING VARIOUS OUTBREAKS

Every year during my tenure at the White House seemed to bring yet another biological threat.

We first heard of severe acute respiratory syndrome (SARS), caused by the SARS-CoV-1 virus (a beta coronavirus), in November 2002. SARS had a major outbreak in China and Canada, with cases continuing through 2003. The initial case fatality rate was reported as 30–40 percent, which is extremely high.

The peak of the SARS contagious period occurs a few days *after* symptoms or fever appear. Estimates suggest that some one thousand deaths occurred worldwide, with thirty-seven other countries reporting cases. Travel management to and from China and Toronto, Canada, became important; Toronto reported at least 257 documented cases (many involving healthcare professionals). While this may have been the first we heard of the coronavirus, it would not be the last.

In 2003 we saw an outbreak of monkeypox, a disease that causes horrific skin lesions. A few cases were detected in the US after victims had traveled from Africa; we believe it came from animals in Ghana. Forty-seven sporadic cases were known, but no sustained human-to-human transmission occurred.

Another outbreak of the disease occurred more recently, beginning in Europe in 2022 and spreading quickly to the Americas and then to all six WHO regions. About eighty-seven thousand cases were reported in one hundred countries, causing 112 deaths. The outbreak affected primarily (but not exclusively) gay men, bisexual men, and other men who had sex with men.[16]

Every September, environmental monitoring in D.C. revealed upticks of tularemia, often right before the annual book fair on the National Mall. The rise in tularemia in monitoring eventually was determined to be related to squirrels, known endemic carriers.

From 2012 to 2015, the beta coronavirus flared up. A type of SARS known as Middle East respiratory syndrome (MERS) resulted in one thousand cases globally and four hundred deaths.

From 2014 to 2015, a severe outbreak of Ebola occurred. Ebola is a deadly, blood-borne viral infection. About twenty-eight thousand cases were reported, with a 70 percent fatality rate, mostly in West Africa but with a few limited cases in Europe and the US.

I was privileged to be part of the transformation of contingency care—that is, providing medical care for special situations. We created plans for smallpox vaccinations and for H1N1, as well as pandemic preparedness for avian influenza.

I also had the opportunity to help change contingency care for category A biological agents and for chemical and radiological agents. In essence, we did what would be expected for zoonotic diseases: prepare for the ongoing care of individuals, with many of the same therapeutics and equipment that make up the national strategic stockpile (including ventilators, personal protective equipment, antidotes, antibiotics, and auto-injectors).

2001 PREPAREDNESS EXERCISES

At the dawn of the millennium, national security agencies conducted an exercise of top officials (TOPOFF) to assess the nation's readiness for a domestic nuclear, biological, or chemical incident. In June 2001, the Department of Defense held an exercise under the name "Dark Winter" featuring scenarios of a smallpox attack on the US population. It shed light on the United States' vulnerability, specifically to smallpox.

Between 2001 and 2003, I participated in several exercises focused on the threat of smallpox. These biodefense preparedness exercises found that more than half of Americans were unvaccinated for the disease. A national strategy was developed to vaccinate the country if indicated. The National Institutes of Health developed a plan that could ramp up vaccine production to fifty-four million doses. It also recommended the possibility of diluting the vaccine up to five times without harming appropriate levels of protection.

I wrote a mass vaccination plan for the Eighteen Acres, which called for shutting down the complex for a day and administering up to five thousand vaccines. The plan never had to be implemented, fortunately, but it was a necessary contingency approach to keep ready in case of human transmission of smallpox anywhere in the world, which would have been considered biological warfare.

THE TRAGEDY OF 9/11

My day started routinely on September 11, 2001, after a weekend off. I was a newbie to the WHMU, scheduled to be the doctor staffing the White House clinic from 9:00 a.m. to 4:00 p.m. Back then, the clinic was located in OEOB, on the first floor in room 105, where it had been since the days of President Nixon.

Before heading to the clinic, I walked through the ground floor of the West Wing. Secret Service agents customarily sit right outside the Situation Room's entrance. On this fateful day, the officer was Scott, whom I had taken care of the week before for some gastrointestinal chest pain. We wore SkyTel pagers, which back then served as primitive precursors to cell phones.

While Scott and I chatted, both our SkyTel pagers went off. The message read, "Small plane hits WTC," referring to the World Trade Center.

"Man," we said, "it must be a bad weather day in New York."

I walked to the White House mess, picked up a cranberry muffin and coffee, and then made my way across West Executive Drive to open the clinic for an ordinary 9:00 a.m. start. On a TV screen there, I saw a scene from New York City . . . on a blue-sky, crystal-clear day.

"Oh, no," I said to myself, "something's up." Just a few moments later, at 9:03 a.m., I watched in disbelief as United Airlines Flight 175 rammed into the South Tower and burst into a gigantic ball of flame.

"Okay," I said, "we're not doing clinic today."

I hurriedly left the clinic with my response bag and headed to the medical unit operations center. A few minutes later, I heard someone say on the Secret Service radio frequency, "Crash at Acrobat," the code name for the Pentagon's landing pad. I looked out from a window and saw smoke rising from the Pentagon. It obviously wasn't a helicopter—I'd spent too much time on military helicopters to confuse a copter crash with whatever this was. We learned later that American Airlines Flight 77 had crashed into the west side of the Pentagon, killing 125 people in the building and all sixty-four passengers on the plane. Security personnel began evacuating the White House and the entire Eighteen Acres.

President Bush wasn't in DC that day; he was in Florida, in a classroom at an elementary school observing their reading program. When the president's security detail whisked him away from Sarasota, however, neither he nor anyone else in his administration knew exactly what was taking place. He was hurriedly escorted to Air Force One, which immediately flew to Barksdale Air Force Base in northwest Louisiana, then later to Offutt Air Force Base just south of Omaha, Nebraska.

Not long after the early morning attacks, the First Lady was moved by her protective detail to an undisclosed location, where she joined the army White House doctor, Dr. Bill Lang. They spent the day there under Secret Service control.

In the chaos of those early hours of 9/11, when President Bush was not immediately accessible, Vice President Cheney gave orders (sometime between 10:12 a.m. and 10:18 a.m.) to shoot down a fourth commercial airliner that radar indicated was heading straight for the White House. He gave the order from the Presidential Emergency Operations Center (PEOC) under the East Wing, where I also headed after learning of the attacks. It was a gutsy call made for the first time in US history.

The vice president, however, is not directly in the chain of military command. If the president is somehow unavailable in an emergency—and he was not always available on that tumultuous morning—the next person in that chain of command is the secretary of defense. But SecDef Donald Rumsfeld was at that time walking outside the Pentagon, viewing damage from the 9:37 a.m. attack. Contrary to official protocol (but an endearing action to those he led), he chose to help rescue the injured still buried in the rubble, which also rendered him not immediately available by phone.

With my blue badge displaying special access, I ran across the north front of the White House through the tradesmen entrance. I made sure I held up my badge and quickly greeted the Secret Service officers now standing out front with their shotguns displayed. "Doc," they responded, "you can go wherever you want. You're on your own."

I ran through the Red Gate, the entrance to the "Marilyn Monroe" tunnel that runs underneath the Executive Mansion. (Back in the 1960s, actress Marilyn Monroe used the tunnel to gain access to the White House for her clandestine visits with President John F. Kennedy.) I entered a bunker under the East Wing called the Presidential Emergency Operations Center (PEOC), a multi-room facility first set up during World War II and greatly expanded during the Cold War. I arrived before Vice President Dick Cheney, who was escorted there by his protective detail. We were joined by National

Security Advisor Condoleezza Rice, White House Communications Director Karen Hughes, Secretary of Transportation Norm Mineta, and other members of the vice president's staff, including his counselor, Mary Matalin. I spent the whole day with them in the bunker, providing medical care and counsel.

My Department of Defense training had taught me that when terrorists attack, they often also launch a more insidious assault. So, at one point, I handed out Cipro (ciprofloxacin, an antibiotic used to fight bacterial infections, often given to those exposed to anthrax or certain types of plague) to some in the PEOC and directed them to take it for a couple of days. Many of them clearly thought I was crazy . . . until three weeks later.

THE ANTHRAX ATTACKS

On October 2, 2001, a photo editor named Robert Stevens contracted anthrax through a letter mailed to him. Several other media outlets and congressional offices had received similar envelopes, also laced with anthrax. The offices of senators Tom Daschle and Patrick Leahy were among those hit, along with some Capitol police officers and staffers of Senator Russ Feingold. Senate offices were shut down for a time to investigate. The multi-week anthrax attacks eventually killed five individuals and infected seventeen others.

The White House has an active staff at the Office of Legislative Affairs. On any given day, about seven thousand people have a badge to work on the Eighteen Acres.

When White House staff were surveyed, a few hundred stated they had been on Capitol Hill on October 9, and therefore potentially exposed. All were surveilled and nasal swabs completed. Fortunately, none of those came back positive for anthrax spores.

After that, no one thought I was crazy. The WHMU staff looked brilliant and could do no wrong.

A full seven years later, DNA evidence led federal prosecutors to name Bruce Edward Ivins as the sole perpetrator of the anthrax attacks. He had worked as a scientist in the biodefense labs at Fort Detrick and committed suicide on July 29, 2008.

AVIAN AND SWINE FLU

The scourge of influenza has played havoc with human populations throughout world history. Many of us know about the great pandemic of 1918, when some fifty million people worldwide died of an influenza outbreak.

Influenza viruses are perpetually present in mammals and birds, and they mutate frequently. In 2003, the strain H5N1, known as avian influenza or bird flu, infected more than seven hundred human individuals, as reported to the World Health Organization. The fifteen countries primarily affected were in Asia, Africa, the Pacific, Europe, and the Middle East. The outbreak eventually spread to sixty other countries. Fortunately, there was no sustained transmission.

Back on October 8, 2001, President Bush had created the Homeland Security Council (HSC) less than a month after 9/11. It became the precursor to today's Department of Homeland Security. In 2005 and 2006, the HSC published the first national strategy preparing for an influenza pandemic. Working with White House planners, I helped develop a pandemic plan for the Eighteen Acres based on the national strategy.

Every modern president makes scores of global trips each year, often visiting places with reported cases of H5N1. We had to make sure we didn't put a traveling team in the path of an influenza outbreak. The antiviral medications, Tamiflu and Relenza, had become popular and got added to the national stockpile.

President Barack Obama was inaugurated in January 2009. An H1N1 swine flu epidemic started in Mexico in April of that year and quickly traveled to the United States. President Obama doubled down on the policies of aggressive vaccine development begun a few years earlier by President Bush. By October 2009, a safe, effective vaccine against H1N1 was in hand, in addition to the quadrivalent seasonal influenza shot.

The CDC estimates that 274,000 H1N1 hospitalizations occurred in the US during 2009, with approximately twelve thousand deaths caused by the virus (estimates range from eight thousand to eighteen thousand). All of us had to learn how to properly use the antiviral medication for those at risk.

South of the border, Mexico had launched its own plan for preparedness. It developed a strategy for surveillance, guidance for how to handle lab specimens, directions for providing various resources for hospitals and medical centers, a strategic reserve of needed medications, and an overall plan for additional public health measures.

In 2007, Mexican president Felipe Calderón had launched a center to identify and keep track of epidemics. Later that year, he established a plan to help government agencies create their own contingency plans for anticipated epidemics and to help them share and coordinate responses.

Between 2004 and 2009, Mexico administered more than eighty thousand influenza vaccines to its citizens, focusing on individuals over the age of fifty and children under the age of three. Mexico also created a strategic reserve of over a million antiviral medications and hundreds of thousands of antibiotics for complicated cases. The country had also created and equipped mobile units and mobile hospitals and secured personal protective equipment, such as protective suits and tens of millions of facemasks.

On January 20, 2009, I began my responsibilities as the physician to the president. On March 18, the disease tracking system in Mexico noticed an increase in the number of respiratory cases throughout the country, consistent with influenza. It was thought to be an extension of the usual seasonal influenza virus, even though the normal winter months had already passed. Nevertheless, an epidemic alert was issued to all health institutions, asking them to assess their preparedness and report any cases of respiratory disease.

Less than two weeks later, on March 28, a nine-year-old girl from Imperial County, California, developed respiratory symptoms.

I was familiar with Imperial County, as I had flown to the naval air facility there in 1986 while doing a rotation with Marine Air Group Thirty-Nine from Camp Pendleton. Soon after the nine-year-old girl reported symptoms, a ten-year-old boy in San Diego reported similar symptoms. The CDC analyzed both cases and identified the virus involved as swine flu, the H1N1 virus.

During the first week in April, I accompanied President Obama on a swing through Europe to attend mini summits. Meanwhile, back in the Americas, more influenza cases were being identified. In the southernmost part of Mexico, in the region of Veracruz, an outbreak had affected a large portion of the community.

President Obama stopped in Iraq for a visit on our way home, arriving back at Andrews Air Force Base (in 2009 the base merged with Naval Air Facility Washington to form Joint Base Andrews) on April 8. Four days later, on April 12, Mexico public health authorities notified the World Health Organization of the outbreak in Veracruz. Samples taken from the Veracruz cases were sent to the CDC, where they were matched to the two cases in Imperial County.

An older lady in Oaxaca City had been hospitalized with pneumonia on April 10; she passed away four days later. Initially, she had been diagnosed with a coronavirus infection, but an autopsy showed that she had the novel H1N1 virus—the first confirmed fatality of the new virus strain.

On April 14, Mexico City reported an unusual number of young patients with severe pneumonia. A White House advance team had been in place there about a week before the president's arrival for a planned visit on April 16. On April 16, the day we landed in Mexico City on official business, Mexico's public health ministry issued an epidemiological alert, reporting an increased number of respiratory cases. Then-current lab capabilities could detect only whether the influenza A virus was present; researchers could not yet identify various strains of the virus.

On the evening of April 16, President Obama took a tour of the National Museum of Anthropology and participated in events outside in the courtyard. I always refer to that event as "night at the museum." The next day, we completed our official visit and returned to Washington, D.C.

About a week after President Obama returned from his Mexico City visit, media outlets began reporting that the curator and director of the National Museum of Anthropology, who had guided President Obama on part of his museum tour, had died. This news suggested that President Obama's health might be in jeopardy.

Because I was familiar with the rapidly evolving H1N1 influenza outbreak in Mexico and in parts of the US, I was asked to look at the case. That meant reviewing a host of complete medical records, which the government of Mexico quickly provided . . . all in Spanish. So, I asked a Spanish-speaking infectious disease consultant from the national medical center to review them.

I soon learned that the sixty-four-year-old gentleman who had died had begun to report upper respiratory symptoms on April 11. He visited his doctor on April 18, the day after the presidential visit. He was hospitalized over the next five days and died of pneumonia, complicated by chronic diseases. The clinical picture clearly was *not* related to viral pneumonia, including influenza. The Associated Press reported this story during the last week of April.

Just before that, on April 20, the CDC published a notice about the discovery of a new strain of the virus. When I reached out to the interim director of the CDC, he asked how he could help. I replied that if he had identified any cases in the Washington, D.C. area, I'd like to know about them. He later told me about two individuals, who I tracked down. Both had been part of the advance team for the president's trip and were appropriately treated with antiviral medication. A week later, I learned that most of the samples were laboratory-confirmed to be the new H1N1 influenza virus.

Back in Mexico, officials immediately suspended classes in the capital. On April 24, President Calderón assumed powers for emergency protection, and on April 27, millions of masks were distributed in

Mexico City. Thirty-seven mobile units were deployed with the capacity to diagnose and treat influenza cases in conjunction with Mexico's national health system.

On April 29, President Calderón addressed his nation in a live TV message. The Mexican federal government closed nonessential government and private sector offices and facilities for the next week.

From the start, Mexican health authorities acted in a timely manner, were responsible, responded quickly based on the information available to them, and mobilized their resources to protect their citizens and visitors. Public health authorities reached out aggressively to their citizens to keep them informed about new developments. The citizens of Mexico responded maturely and with a strong sense of responsibility, which helped to curtail the H1N1 influenza outbreak there.

Later that year, as noted, a vaccine for the novel strain of the H1N1 virus became widely available. Health officials recommended that women and children get their shots first. After the District of Columbia recommended the shot for healthy adult males, President Obama was among the first to roll up his sleeve, not out of concern for himself, but as an example to others in the community and around the nation that he put his faith in this safe, effective vaccine.

LIFE EXPERIENCE PREPARES YOU

I've learned many things from my medical career and time at the White House, and one of them is that life experience can prepare a person for what lies ahead. I believe that my time in the military and at the WHMU prepared me for the COVID-19 pandemic of 2019–2022 and enabled me to contribute to an effective response to it through my current work at AdventHealth.

During my military career, I had learned much from the Department of Defense's Medical Management of Chemical, Biological, and Radiological Casualties course; at the Aberdeen Proving Ground for chemical agents; at Fort Detrick for biological agents; and had spent lots of time learning from general advisers in chemical and biological warfare.

I also had spent time with Homeland Security on preparedness; interacted with members of the National Security Council; learned from the CDC's Epidemiological Intelligence Service; observed the Emergency Operations Center; spoken with a forward-deployed virologist; and had discussions with global migration medical experts around the world.

Medically speaking, you never know what lies ahead, but blithely believing that whatever has protected you in the past will continue to do so is simply unwise.

I'm a navy guy, not a member of the US Coast Guard, but I nevertheless love the Coast Guard's motto: *Semper Paratus*—always ready.

Indeed.

10

CABINET CARE

All US presidents get to designate qualified individuals to become part of their administration to serve as members of the cabinet. Cabinet members often work as the secretaries or the leaders of specific governmental or military agencies, such as the secretary of defense, secretary of state, White House chief of staff, director of the CIA, and attorney general.

In the past couple of decades, healthcare provided by the government for these individuals has greatly expanded. In my view, it only makes sense to extend the principle of "care by proxy" to the men and women who wield such great influence in every presidential administration, since some of them, such as the vice president or the secretary of defense, are in a direct line of succession to the highest office in the land.

But just as it took some time for presidential healthcare to evolve to its current state, it also took some time for cabinet care to develop at all. It may be that one factor prompting this evolution was the assassination of President John F. Kennedy and the chaos and blurred lines of responsibilities that immediately followed.

AN AUTOPSY FOR THE PRESIDENT

One day after I made a presentation at the Mayo Clinic, a man approached and told me that he was in one of two ambulances that met Air Force One when the plane carrying the body of the slain president landed at Andrews Air Force Base. One ambulance had arrived to take the body to the Walter Reed Army Medical Center for an autopsy, while the second ambulance had come to take the president's remains to Bethesda Naval Hospital for the same autopsy. The two groups had a heated argument and eventually the body ended up going to the navy hospital at Bethesda.

The argument arose primarily because no procedure had been established ahead of time for such a tragic event. Walter Reed was originally the US Army hospital, while Bethesda was established as the US Navy hospital. Since President Kennedy had served in the navy during World War II as the commander of PT-109, the Bethesda ambulance crew had a fierce loyalty to one of their own.

To this day, accusations fly of a botched autopsy at Bethesda. The body should have gone to Walter Reed, some say, because the staff there was much more experienced and better equipped for the critical procedure. And hence, the argument goes, conspiracy theories about JFK's assassination continue to multiply when they could have been eliminated by an autopsy performed by those best trained to do it. But since no policy existed to give direction in such a chaotic situation, those with the loudest and most passionate voices prevailed.

Because none of us know what's going to happen tomorrow, three hours from now, or even in the next minute, it makes sense to have procedures and resources in place to ensure (as much as possible) the continuity of the presidency and the smooth functioning of the government. Care by proxy maintains that by taking better care of those who serve the president, we take better care of the president and, by extension, better care of the nation itself.

A Short History of Cabinet Care

Government-provided healthcare of cabinet members is based on a historical arrangement called the secretarial designee program. The secretary of one of the armed forces—the secretary of the navy, for example—may designate that certain individuals not on active duty or who are not otherwise eligible beneficiaries of Department of Defense care, can, even so, receive care at a military treatment facility.

On May 23, 1968, the secretary of the navy (SECNAV) designated that former First Family members would have access to healthcare. This decision allowed former First Family members, such as Jacqueline Kennedy, to receive care at a military treatment facility. The family members of former president Eisenhower already were eligible beneficiaries.

Fifteen years later, on November 23, 1983, SECNAV designated the president, vice president, and four-star equivalent civilian leaders to be eligible to receive care at military treatment facilities. A few months after that, on April 27, 1984, the rule was clarified to say that this directive included the president, vice president, and members of the cabinet.

Almost a decade later, on October 28, 1993, a second navy council clarified the definition of "current First Family members" who could be eligible for care at a military treatment facility. That June, the president announced that First Family members would be eligible for care at a military treatment facility. The next year, SECNAV, as per the Bureau of Medicine and Surgery (BUMED), directed and expanded this designation to include vice presidents and their immediate families. In March 1996, SECNAV restated that this provision included the president, the vice president, and members of the president's cabinet. And on January 5, 2004, the secretary of defense added assistants to the president and the director of the White House Military Office to be included in the secretarial designee program.

The architecture at Bethesda was inspired by hand drawings of FDR, so it seems appropriate that a medical evaluation treatment unit for the care of US presidents has operated there as far back as President Kennedy. Care of the president formerly took place at the historic Walter Reed hospital or Bethesda. Back then, Walter Reed had the Eisenhower Executive Suite (Eisenhower was an army general). President Eisenhower always went to the army hospital, Walter Reed, but since President Kennedy was navy, he had allegiance to Bethesda.

CARE FOR THE FIRST FAMILY

While no black-and-white rules exist for the medical care of the First Family, we do have historical, legal, and practical precedence.

We took much of our guidance from the Secret Service Protection Act (18 United States Code 3056) and the Secretarial Designation Program (32 CFR Part 728). We had additional guidance from HIPAA (the Health Insurance Portability and Accountability Act of 1996 that restricts access to individuals' private medical information), from the Joint Commission, and similar accrediting agencies. We made sure that everyone had the proper credentials and the required professional privileges through Bethesda or Walter Reed.

We worked hard to provide private, secure access to top quality care to eligible beneficiaries. If that care took the form of military medicine or healthcare provided by the WHMU, no fees were charged. If they received outpatient care in the national capital region at a military treatment facility, the fee was waived, while inpatient care (hospital overnight admission) was billed at interagency rates, per regulations.

We had to complete secretarial designation for each First Family member and keep that information up to date, following the rules of engagement. For the First Family, if civilian medical or dental care was coordinated by the physician to the president, the civilian providers would bill their services to insurance, making sure to follow all appropriate rules.

It takes a network to provide healthcare at the White House, and usually, that care is geared toward individual patients. We established a nexus of care through the WHMU. The beauty of being the president of the United States is that the physician to the president takes care of all that for you and your family.

Military and civilian hospitals in the Washington D.C. area, along with their medical specialty consultants, provided the main network of care. Those centers included Walter Reed, the National Institutes of Health, George Washington University Hospital, Georgetown, Inova, MedStar, Johns Hopkins, and Shock Trauma at the University of Maryland Medical Center.

At the White House itself, the doctor's office was located on the ground floor of the Executive Residence. A procedure exam room connects to it, able to be quickly configured to provide the day-to-day care that the president or First Family might need.

Another full-service clinic was located on the ground floor of the OEOB. Still another medical facility was perpetually equipped and ready at Eucalyptus, a cabin located on the grounds of Camp David. We also had medical capabilities at the president's official "second residence" aboard Air Force One, as well as globally wherever the president and his entourage would travel.

Access to a dentist is incredibly important. Dental care was provided by the dean of the Naval Postgraduate Dental School at Walter Reed. During my time at the White House, Captain (Dr.) Glenn Munro did an incredible job of leading his team. We also had access to orthodontics, oral surgery, periodontics, and whatever other dental care might be required. A full dental chair and operatory stood ready in the basement of the White House.

Optometry is equally important. I helped set up an eye lane at the OEOB. We used the Department of Defense program called Frames of Choice, and if the individual wanted contacts, those had to be purchased privately. Aaron Tarbett, OD, was the gifted optometrist who cared for the president, First Family, and set up the first eye lane on the Eighteen Acres.

EXPANDING CABINET CARE

In 2001, as part of the White House Medical Unit Executive Medicine Program, I established Cabinet Care, as allowable by law and regulations. We conceived it as a program to provide comprehensive, confidential, and accessible medical services to cabinet members who served as the president's most senior advisors. The goal of the Executive Medicine Program was to provide healthcare while maximizing the availability, performance, and efficiency of cabinet members.

A healthy team is essential to a strong performing administration. We provided our services 365 days a year, both at home and abroad. The executive medical services included a periodic executive physical, which we performed at Walter Reed or Bethesda Naval. Travel medicine included medical advice, destination-specific immunizations, medications, and self-aid medical kits. It also included primary care to treat chronic conditions, as well as acute care and advice for minor illnesses and injuries that might occur at the office, at home, or during travel.

For specialty care regarding more complex medical issues that we could not effectively manage in the White House Medical Clinic, we arranged a referral to medical or surgical specialists elsewhere. We also provided support to deliver prescription medications to be filled at hospital-based military pharmacies, maintaining secure medical records in accordance with HIPAA. Those medical records were to return to cabinet members at the end of their tenure in office or transferred to the medical office they authorized. We provided protective medical support as well for those who were part of the designated successor programs, enacted in accordance with continuity procedures.

Medical coverage provided to the vice president of the United States, as the designated successor to the president, shifted in 2001 from sporadic care during official duties to round-the-clock care, 24/7/365. This was fortuitous, as Vice President Cheney, who had excellent care from his cardiologist at George Washington University, kept the WHMU busy with his extensive domestic and global travel.

By the time of this change in cabinet medical coverage, he already had a long history of chronic health conditions, especially coronary heart disease. He had his first heart attack (of five) in 1978 at the age of thirty-seven and underwent quadruple bypass surgery ten years later. A White House physician and a military aide from one of the five military services made sure they provided round-the-clock coverage for the vice president as the designated successor.

DEAD BODIES ON THE WHITE HOUSE GROUNDS

You might find the question gruesome, but what happens when someone finds a dead body on the White House grounds? It happens more than you might think, just as it does at hotels all around the world.

When I discovered that we had no plan to address such situations, I also realized we had a problem. Who takes charge in such an event? The Capitol Police? The US military? The Secret Service? The D.C. police force? I understood that if we wanted to avoid a clash of authorities reminiscent of what happened in 1963 regarding the body of President Kennedy, we needed a plan to follow. The plot of the 1997 movie *Murder at 1600* depicts the tensions between the Secret Service and Metropolitan police over jurisdiction and methods.

And so, I developed the following two algorithms.

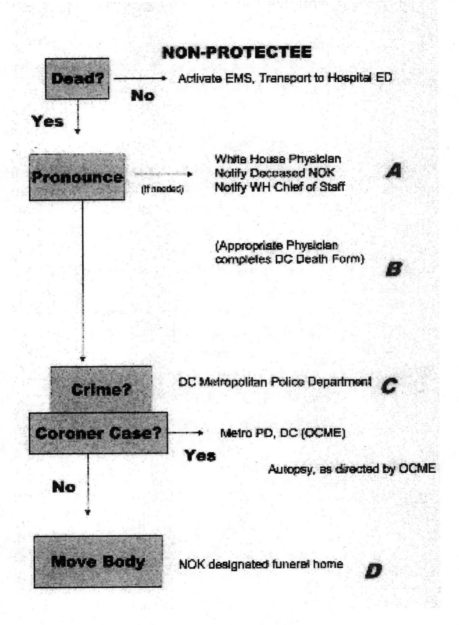

NON-PROTECTEE

Dead? → Activate EMS, Transport to Hospital ED

No

Yes

Pronounce → White House Physician
Notify Deceased NOK
Notify WH Chief of Staff **A**
(If needed)

(Appropriate Physician completes DC Death Form) **B**

Crime? DC Metropolitan Police Department **C**

Coroner Case? → Metro PD, DC (OCME)
Yes

Autopsy, as directed by OCME

No

Move Body NOK designated funeral home **D**

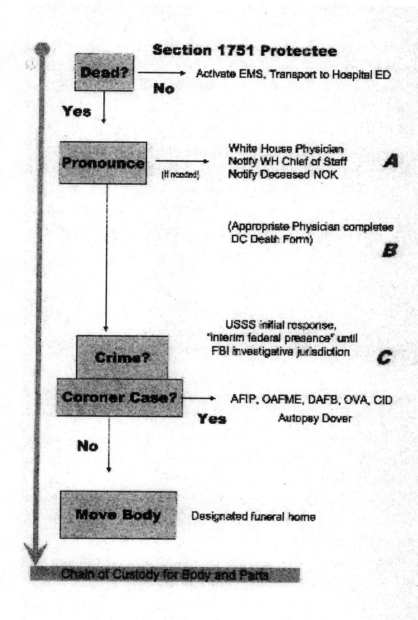

Section 1751 Protectee

Dead? → Activate EMS, Transport to Hospital ED

No

Yes

Pronounce → White House Physician
(If needed) Notify WH Chief of Staff
Notify Deceased NOK   A

(Appropriate Physician completes
DC Death Form)   B

USSS initial response,
"interim federal presence" until
FBI investigative jurisdiction   C

Crime?

Coroner Case? → AFIP, OAFME, DAFB, OVA, CID
Yes   Autopsy Dover

No

Move Body   Designated funeral home

Chain of Custody for Body and Parts

The healthy discussions and table-top exercises leading up to the algorithms were critical to identifying the proper roles of the White House physician or law enforcement in such an event. Fortunately, we never had to pull out the algorithms during my tenure.

We determined that the notification of next of kin would fall to the White House chief of staff or their designee. For the determination of a possible crime scene, initial response and security would be the responsibility of the Secret Service as the interim federal presence until the FBI arrives and assumes investigative jurisdiction. For coroner cases, the Armed Forces Institute of Pathology's Office of the Armed Forces Medical Examiner, located on Dover Air Force Base, would be expected to work in conjunction with the FBI's Criminal Investigative Division. Once those investigations conclude, the remains would go to the mortuary of the next of kin's choosing.

BOTH WISE AND NECESSARY

One of the first cabinet members for whom I had the privilege of helping negotiate healthcare in D.C. was Condoleezza Rice. In 2001, Dr. Rice was the first woman appointed to be the national security advisor. Later, during President Bush's second administration, she became the first African American woman to serve as secretary of state.

She has a remarkable life story, playing as a pianist with the Denver Symphony Orchestra at age fifteen and enrolling at the University of Denver at age sixteen. She soon switched majors from music performance to international studies and received her bachelor's degree at age nineteen. A year later, she completed a master's degree at Notre Dame, and in 1981, at age twenty-six, she earned a PhD from the University of Denver.

Although she never played professionally as a concert pianist, she did play occasionally in public, a couple of times with cellist Yo-Yo Ma and then also at an embassy function for Queen Elizabeth II.

Dr. Rice was young, healthy, and physically fit. After she moved from Stanford University, where she had served as provost for six years, she needed some help coordinating her routine medical care in D.C. At one point I accompanied her to Walter Reed, where we had scheduled a routine physical for her. When she told me she was having some issues with wrist pain, I asked how often she played the piano. She reported that she practiced on her Steinway one hour every day.

"That seems like a lot to me," I said.

"Oh, no," she replied, "I used to practice four hours a day."

As we spoke, the president tracked her down and asked what she was doing. When she replied that she was getting a routine physical, he replied, "Oh, sorry to bother you. I'm glad you're getting that done," and quickly let her get back to her business.

That little incident reminded me that cabinet members have many pressing issues continually on their plates. They must be able to take care of personal medical issues expeditiously and efficiently, coordinated by a physician familiar with the various options for their care. In the modern era, cabinet care is not only wise but also a necessity.

11

The Physical and Mental Requirements to Be President

The responsibilities of the physician to the president have greatly broadened over the past two decades. Four major areas of healthcare for the president have permanently changed, or been transformed, since the beginning of the twenty-first century:

1. The concept of "Care Under Fire": The physician to the president is better prepared for penetrating trauma (gunshots or knife stabbings) with the principles, equipment, and training of Tactical Combat Casualty Care.

2. Asymmetrical threats: The physician to the president is better prepared, equipped, and trained to expertly care for chemical and biological threats, including pandemics.

3. Global travel: The physician to the president has adopted the idea of providing care "anywhere and everywhere,"

including on Air Force One or Marine One, in motorcade vehicles (e.g., limousines, ambulances, and "Linebacks"— SUVs that carry the protective detail shift), or on the Eighteen Acres (White House residence, West Wing, East Wing, Executive Office Building, or other locations), at Camp David, and in the president's second residence(s).

4. Whole person care: The physician to the president optimizes their patients' fitness and integrates care to address the needs of the mind, body, and spirit.

Another important responsibility emerging in the last decade is what I call "evaluation of critical decision-making." That's the chief issue we'll investigate in this chapter; but before we do so, let's consider the constitutional requirements for serving as the president of the United States.

THE PRESIDENT AND THE CONSTITUTION

The Constitution, written in the late eighteenth century, describes the role and the required qualifications of the president of the United States. It states that for an individual to qualify for the office of president, the person must be at least thirty-five years of age, be a natural-born citizen, and have lived in the US for at least fourteen years.

And that's it.

The requirement to be a natural-born citizen has long been debated by constitutional scholars. Does it mean someone who is born an American citizen, even if born elsewhere? Or does it refer to an American citizen born on US soil, including its territories? Or that the individual must be someone born within the borders of a US state? The first few presidents, in fact, were born as British subjects.

This requirement is likely to be tested in the coming years, but we already have theoretical examples to ponder from our recent past. Consider, for example, the late senator John McCain, who was born to US military personnel serving in the Panama Canal zone. Would he have qualified to become a US president, according to the Constitution?

THE TWENTY-FIFTH AMENDMENT

In the aftermath of the assassination of John F. Kennedy in November 1963, the Twenty-Fifth Amendment was proposed in 1965 and ratified by the required number of states on February 10, 1967. Consider the first three of its four sections:

> *Section 1*
> In case of the removal of the President from office or of his death or resignation, the Vice President shall become President.

> *Section 2*
> Whenever there is a vacancy in the office of the Vice President, the President shall nominate a Vice President who shall take office upon confirmation by a majority vote of both Houses of Congress.

> *Section 3*
> Whenever the President transmits to the President pro tempore of the Senate and the Speaker of the House of Representatives his written declaration that he is unable to discharge the powers and duties of his office, and until he transmits to them a written declaration to the contrary, such powers and duties shall be discharged by the Vice President as Acting President.

We have a long list of examples throughout American history regarding presidential deaths and disability, whether natural or unnatural (see chapter 1). A disability could be either temporary or permanent.

A personal example of a temporary impairment that prompted a US president to voluntarily turn over the authority of his office occurred in June 2002. At that time, President George W. Bush underwent a scheduled colonoscopy at Camp David. I had briefed the president about the procedure and prep while onboard Air Force One, as we flew home from a G8 summit in Kananaskis, Canada. The president cheekily asked if Dr. Butler, the gastroenterologist scheduled to do the procedure, was a rear admiral.

"Only if you promote him," I answered.

In 2002, colonoscopies were typically done under conscious sedation using a combination of narcotics and benzodiazepine, rendering the patient groggy for the rest of the day. "Don't operate any heavy equipment or make any important decisions," went the standard advice from the doctor performing the sedation. The chairman at Bethesda Naval insisted on Demerol and Valium. I was up on the literature, discussed the procedure with expert anesthesiologists, and even called the leaders of the American Society of Anesthesiologists, who instead all advocated for propofol (a.k.a. "milk of amnesia") under the constant, strict monitoring of an anesthesiologist bedside during the procedure.

The president cited Section 3 of the Twenty-Fifth Amendment when he signed a piece of paper on a corpsmen's wooden desk at the Eucalyptus Cabin, thereby temporarily turning over the duties of president to Vice President Dick Cheney for the next two or three hours. Cheney was considered the acting president for that time, while President Bush underwent propofol general anesthesia. During that period, Mr. Bush appropriately gave over the duties of the US president to Vice President Cheney. The entire presidential support apparatus shifted to Acting President Cheney during that time.

We faxed the form to Congress while the original document was driven down to the Capitol and delivered in person. For the next couple of hours after the procedure, the president walked his dog and chatted with Josh Bolten, his deputy chief of staff. The effects of anesthesia had not only completely worn off, but multiple chemical deterioration half-lives also had passed. When the president under-went examination by the White House physician and specialists, they determined he was 100 percent back to normal, and so he took back the full powers of the presidency and lifted the temporary granting of presidential powers. That's a perfect example of Section 3 of the Twenty-Fifth Amendment in action.

Such a procedure has clear guidelines, which by tradition are carried by the physician to the president in their duty medical bag. Interestingly, however, Section 3 of the Twenty-Fifth Amendment mentions nothing about a physician.

SECTION 4 OF THE TWENTY-FIFTH AMENDMENT

Section 4 of the Twenty-Fifth Amendment has never been put into action. It reads as follows:

Section 4
Whenever the Vice President and a majority of either the principal officers of the executive departments or of such other body as Congress may by law provide, transmit to the President pro tempore of the Senate and the Speaker of the House of Representatives their written declaration that the President is unable to dis-charge the powers and duties of his office, the Vice President shall immediately assume the powers and duties of the office as Acting President.

Thereafter, when the President transmits to the President pro tempore of the Senate and the Speaker of the House of Representatives his written declaration that no inability exists, he shall resume the powers and duties of his office unless the Vice President and a ma-jority of either the principal officers of the executive de-partment or of such other body as Congress may by law provide, transmit within four days to the President pro tempore of the Senate and the Speaker of the House of Representatives their written declaration that the President is unable to discharge the powers and duties of his office. Thereupon Congress shall decide the issue, assembling within forty-eight hours for that purpose if not in session. If the Congress, within twenty-one days after receipt of the latter written declaration, or, if Congress is not in session, within twenty-one days after Congress is required to assemble, determines by two-thirds vote of both Houses that the President is unable to discharge the powers and duties of his office, the Vice President shall continue to discharge the same as Acting President; otherwise, the President shall resume the powers and duties of his office.

Section 4 concerns the *involuntary* suspension of the president's powers and duties when the president can no longer carry them out. It involves the president's cabinet, the vice president, and a very specific process for invoking such an involuntary suspension of powers.

Senator Birch Bayh, who wrote the section, used the word "inability" and the phrase "unable to discharge the powers and duties of his office" to describe a situation in which a sitting president came to lack the ability to function as president. Senator Bayh may have had in mind, primarily, a person lacking the mental capacity to function as president.

What kind of physical impairments could trigger the implementation of Section 4? First, let's consider some basic definitions.

An "impairment" is a medical or physical condition in which the person is not 100 percent able to perform a specific function. Examples might include a hearing impairment or a visual impairment, or if someone had limited use of an arm or a leg. All of those are impairments.

A second word that comes into play is "accommodation," which refers to something that can be put in place to mitigate partially or fully the identified impairment. If the impairment is hearing, a hearing

JEFFREY KUHLMAN, MD, MPH

aid might be the accommodation. If the impairment is a broken leg, a crutch or wheelchair might be the accommodation.

The third critical term is "disability." A disability is declared based on an administrative judgment regarding that specific impairment and the proposed accommodation. Is it reasonable or unreasonable? Is it practical? Does the specified impairment, along with the proposed accommodation, amount to a disability? These are not strictly *constitutional* questions, for as we have seen, the US Constitution states only the president must be a natural-born citizen of the United States, be at least thirty-five years old, and have been a resident of the United States for fourteen years. It mandates no other physical or mental requirements.

Almost all physical impairments can be reasonably accommodated. We have had multiple presidents with hearing, visual, and even ambulatory impairments. The one impairment that cannot be accommodated is the ability to make critical decisions. When presented with a complex problem, can the individual analyze the information and render a coherent directive?

A fourth concept is "administrative decision." The president must be able to do certain things to get the job done. The office of president is filled by the electoral college, based on the votes of each state. The American people get the president they elect. Presidential campaigns provide American voters with ample information to decide who is qualified for the job. You could think of this as something like a pre-employment physical.

WHAT MIGHT TRIGGER SECTION 4?

The Twenty-Fifth Amendment provides fodder for politicians or pundits to make sound bites against current or future leaders. Unless and until we come to a time when Section 4 of the Twenty-Fifth Amendment is invoked, it may be difficult to envision what such a situation might look like.

We can, of course, find some Hollywood examples of something like it—the 1993 film *Dave* comes to mind—but Section 4 has never yet been invoked in American history. Tom Clancy also imagined what an out-of-the-ordinary presidential succession might look like in a series of techno-thrillers built on one another (*The Sum of All Fears*, 1991; *Debt of Honor*, 1994; *Executive Orders*, 1996). What might the implementation of Section 4 look like if it were to be invoked sometime in the future?

Imagine a devastating, hemorrhagic stroke that rendered the president unconscious and lying in a long-term coma. Other medical conditions, such as severe dementia, major (Axis I) psychiatric disorders, massive trauma, and terminal brain cancer, could also trigger Section 4. Medical experts, likely including the physician to the president, would provide medical information and guidance based on evaluations to the cabinet (the vice president and principal officers of the executive departments), who could then make a written declaration to the president pro tempore of the Senate and the Speaker of the House stating that the president was unable to discharge the powers and duties of the office. The vice president would then immediately assume the powers and duties of the office as *acting* president.

For such an unprecedented scenario in such unchartered waters, we would have to wait to see what unfolds. Something not explicitly specified in Section 4 of the Twenty-Fifth Amendment could take place. Could the vice president continue to serve as acting president until the next election cycle? Maybe.

Let's hope we never find out.

THE VOTERS DECIDE

To win the job of president of the United States, an individual must convince the American people that he/she has the wherewithal to do the job. That determination is up to eligible voters who participate in the general election.

And yet, in the twenty-first century, only a tiny portion of us ever meet the presidential candidates in person. Nevertheless, all of us have an opportunity to watch the candidates on television, online, or in different multimedia events. We can see how they talk. We get glimpses into how they think. We observe how they speak, how they write, the executive function they display, and their temperament. At this moment in history, we have more information than ever about the candidates running for the highest office in our nation.

Once a candidate is elected and takes office, we see how they function during the next four years. When they attend world summits of global leaders, are they passive or do they actively engage and participate? Do they lead the events? Do they spur new thinking? Do they effectively address the nation? Do they hold regular, informative news conferences? How do they deliver prepared remarks? How do they handle off-the-cuff remarks? How do they interact with speech writers? How do they appear to treat those around them and those who work with and for them? *All* of that is a matter of both public and private record.

Voters get to decide if the parties' candidates appear to have the mental capacity to serve as president. As voters, *we* make that choice. Once the president-elect has been inaugurated and taken the oath of office, then that individual remains president until he/she finishes the four-year term, dies, resigns, or is removed.

AGE AND CRITICAL DECISION-MAKING

How can we tell if a president has suffered such a significant loss in the critical decision-making function that he or she ought to be removed from office through the invocation of Section 4 of the Twenty-Fifth Amendment? Some obvious things that could significantly cloud a president's judgment might include:

- impairment caused by certain medications;
- alcohol, including both acute and chronic abuse;
- a diagnosed Axis I psychiatric condition as characterized in the fifth edition of the *Diagnostic and Statistical Manual of Mental Disorders* (the *DSM-5*); and/or
- severe cognitive decline, such as dementia (a progressive, accelerated mental disability due to a neurodegenerative condition).

Normal aging individuals have minimal or mild cognitive decline. You would not expect severe cognitive decline unless they have dementia or another pathology. Of the first forty-four presidents, the oldest on record at the time of inauguration was Ronald Reagan. When he was inaugurated, President Reagan was sixty-nine years old; he served as president for eight years. The youngest to become president was Teddy Roosevelt, who was forty-two when he took office on September 14, 1901, after the assassination of President William McKinley.

In this regard I cannot avoid mentioning the 2024 election. If things continue to move in the same direction as they appear to be headed now, on election day, the candidate of one major party will be seventy-eight. That age is the oldest in American presidential history. It's often said that age, in and of itself, is just a number. But in fact, it's not just the age—it's the mileage.

When people talk about their concerns regarding a candidate's age, it's not precisely the age that concerns them, but rather the condition and performance of the body and the effects on the mind that typically come with advancing age. Sometimes elderly people have gait disturbances; they lack the good balance they once enjoyed. They also have decreased mobility, with less flexibility of the spine and less mobility of the joints. Those conditions are typical of the physical decline that tends to come with each advancing year.

The term "executive functioning" refers to an individual engaging in independent, appropriate, purposeful behavior, including the ability to engage in appropriate self-care. Cognitive abilities include the ability to self-monitor, plan, problem-solve, organize, reason, and remain mentally flexible.

Research has shown that concept formation, abstraction, and mental flexibility all tend to decline with age, especially after age seventy.[17] Older adults tend to think more concretely than younger adults. Aging also negatively affects response inhibition, the ability to restrain an automatic response in favor of producing a novel response.[18] Reasoning with unfamiliar material also declines with age.

Humans' cognitive ability (memory, reasoning, spatial visualization, speed) possibly peaks out in their mid-twenties. When we move past age sixty, the average person's cognitive decline accelerates. Consider the following from the archives of the National Institute on Aging:

- "Relatively little decline in performance occurs until people are about 50 years old."[19]
- "Most abilities tend to peak in early midlife, plateau until the late fifties or sixties, and then show decline, initially at a slow pace, but accelerating as the late seventies are reached."[20]
- "Cognitive abilities generally remain stable throughout adult life until around age sixty."[21]
- "Cognitive decline may begin after midlife, but most often occurs at higher ages (70 or higher)."[22]
- "No or little drop in performance before age 55."[23]
- "Age-related cognitive decline begins relatively early in adulthood . . . the magnitude of age-related decline accelerates (2–4x) at older ages (61–96 years of age)."[24]

Increasing age is the highest known risk factor for cognitive impairment. Cardiovascular risk factors such as diabetes, high blood pressure, and high cholesterol, along with depression, physical frailty, low education levels, and low social support levels, also are associated with a greater risk of cognitive impairment.

In normal aging, cognitive performance, such as executive function or decision-making, processing speed, and recall or retrieval of information may slow down, but the changes are subtle and distinctly different.

Dementia is a neurodegenerative condition with greater cognitive decline than is caused by normal aging. The most common cause of dementia is Alzheimer's disease. Dementia may include problems with language, disorientation, extreme mood swings, loss of motivation, self-neglect, and behavioral issues. An individual's cognitive impairment may not be severe enough to interfere with the functions of independent activities. Some people with mild cognitive impairment progress to dementia, but many do not.

What is the difference between forgetfulness and dementia? If an individual can't remember where they put their keys, that is memory recall failure or forgetfulness. If an individual is shown a set of car keys and doesn't know what they are or what they are used for, that is dementia.

Does an episode of confusion, memory lapse, or verbal stumbling reflect or foreshadow serious mental decline? Experts don't easily know. Fatigue, a recent concussive event, medications, and transient vascular events can confuse any snapshot in time. Comprehensive tests that are hours long and administered by trained experts can evaluate language skills, executive function, problem-solving, spatial skills, attentiveness, and different types of memory.

A physician or a spouse who has known the individual for many years is in a prime position to assess a change in cognitive function over time. Testing done on an individual, compared to comparable testing done five to ten years prior, can also be helpful, though it is rarely available.

When asked by a family to assess a loved one, a primary care doctor uses a validated screening tool. The most common tools are the Mini-Mental Status Examination (MMSE) or the Montreal Cognitive Assessment (MoCA).

The MMSE is a thirty-point questionnaire covering orientation, naming objects, spelling words, counting backward, recalling words, and following standardized tasks. A lower score may indicate dementia but is never diagnostic. The MMSE is not sensitive to (has no ability to diagnose) mild cognitive impairment or early dementia and requires the tested individual to have a certain level of education, which most presidents have. A score of twenty-four to thirty is consistent with normal cognition and no dementia. Unfortunately, if an individual misses one point, although clinically meaningless, the political opposition would pounce.

MoCA, according to medical literature, is more sensitive to the early detection of mild cognitive impairment. MoCA involves tests for short-term memory, executive functions, visuospatial abilities, language, and orientation to time and place, as well as attention, concentration, and working memory. MoCA also has a thirty-point maximum and takes about ten minutes.

There is no requirement for cognitive screening to be part of a presidential physical. President Trump completed the MoCA test in 2018 and scored thirty out of thirty, as reported by the physician to the president at the time, Dr. Ronny Jackson. Dr. Jackson stated that he did not believe it was clinically indicated to take the test, but the president had insisted on it. At the time, certain media coverage and commentary questioned the president's mental fitness for office. The MoCA can screen for mild cognitive impairment or dementia, which clearly Mr. Trump didn't have, but it does not screen or test for other aspects of mental fitness or other neuropsychiatric conditions. My professional opinion is that the MoCA of thirty was accurate and consistent with the president's public mental abilities at that time.

A review of the literature shows that about a third of people with mild cognitive impairment develop dementia in the next five years. The same studies, however, also show that about a third of people with mild cognitive impairment may return to their normal cognition over five years.[25] It is also important to note that approximately 10 percent of individuals with dementia evaluated by a medical professional have an identified cause that is reversible.[26]

TOO OLD TO RULE?

When is it too old to rule? It's not just one of the leading parties' 2024 candidate for president who is the oldest in history and therefore an extreme outlier. We also have the oldest Congress in history. For the House of Representatives in the 118th Congress, half of our representatives are baby boomers or, even older, members of the Silent Generation, born before 1945.

On the Senate side, it's even more pronounced, with seventy-three of our one hundred senators being boomers or members of that Silent Generation, the oldest contingent of Americans.

If you think back to 1776 in the colonies and then for the next one hundred years in the United States, Americans had a life expectancy in the mid-thirties. We know that was tamped down low by infant and childhood mortality, but overall life expectancy remained in the mid-thirties until three-quarters of the way through the nineteenth century. In 1850, if you made it to age ten, your life expectancy was well into your fifties. Today, life expectancy is in the mid-seventies (the average is about seventy-seven years). Of course, that life expectancy is calculated from a person's birth. A different life expectancy would apply to someone who has reached eighty years of age.

So, what are we afraid of? Every year that we age, our physical and mental function changes. We may gain some wisdom, but our cognitive function declines over time, although that decline varies widely among individuals.

If you take all Americans aged seventy-five to eighty-four, only 13 percent have dementia. That means that 87 percent do *not* have dementia. They may be normal functioning or they may have some mild cognitive impairment, but 87 percent of Americans aged seventy-five to eighty-four do not have dementia (data provided by the Alzheimer's Association, which keeps a close tab on these functions).

As physicians, we are often asked to weigh in on this issue when a loved one gets older. We have a saying in medicine that once you've seen one eighty-year-old, you've seen one eighty-year-old. Each individual case is different. I think of my dad.

My father is a member of the Silent Generation, those born before World War II (he was born in 1939). He is a PhD-trained nuclear physicist who studied at Purdue University in the 1960s. He is still teaching at age eighty-five, and he is not teaching merely general education courses like earth science or astronomy, or even general physics, to pre-med students. He's taught some of those courses, but more often he teaches the difficult, calculus-based, upper division, university-level engineering and physics courses of statics and dynamics. In addition, he routinely tutors students in Calculus 1, Calculus 2, and differential equations. His students now include his twenty-one grandchildren.

Every day he demonstrates his neurocognitive ability. One professor new to the university audited his class as part of succession planning. He asked my eighty-five-year-old father for additional help and tutoring in some of the more difficult concepts.

My dad is on top of his game. If you ask him, he'll say, "Not a lot has changed in nuclear physics in the last sixty years." A cognitive decline screening test certainly could be done for him, but it would be completely useless. And it is not clinically indicated.

In general, however, as our brain ages, bits and pieces of our memory start to drop out. We forget some things, perhaps so that we can remember other things. We don't really have the option of expanding our storage. Forgetting a name, occasionally choosing the wrong term, misplacing car keys—those are certainly a common part of normal aging. Sometimes we forget due to distraction, and at other times, we simply have a memory lapse.

We live in an age when more Americans than ever are working well past their seventies. In healthcare, we have doctors, surgeons, and nurses who fit in that category. The chief clinical officer of our large healthcare system is seventy-five years old and remains as sharp as ever, fully engaged in all the current concepts. He'll tell you he doesn't have the stamina that he did a few decades ago, but his cognitive ability has not declined. I also think of at least three surgeons I know who are working into their nineties and still doing a great job.

But that's certainly not true for every surgeon. Some hospitals and healthcare systems, therefore, have enacted "Aging Surgeon Programs" in which these surgeons are taken through one or two days of testing, not just of their cognitive ability but also of their physical skills. To be a surgeon or nurse, often you must use your hands. You must have good eye coordination and good visual acuity so that the movement of your hands matches what you're trying to do. Some medical functions are highly technically oriented.

An Aging Surgeon Program usually takes a multidisciplinary approach, where physical therapists, occupational therapists, physicians, and administrative experts in ethics and legal practice all weigh in. Surgeons get an objective evaluation. Healthcare would benefit from picking an age, maybe starting at age seventy-five, for all surgeons to begin getting tested every couple of years.

Another front is the law. The Age Discrimination in Employment Act became the law of the land in 1967 and forbids mandatory age-related retirement at age 70 for many jobs. The law does allow exceptions when public safety is involved. For example, FBI agents are forced to retire as agents at age fifty-seven. That job does have a large physical component in addition to a mental one. Commercial airline transport pilots have a mandatory retirement at age sixty-five. A program that would allow individuals to demonstrate their physical and mental abilities could keep individuals in either profession working longer, to everyone's benefit.

UNDIAGNOSED NEUROPSYCHIATRIC CONDITIONS

While conditions like those just discussed can severely impair the critical thinking and decision-making functions of a president, senator, or congressperson, they do not exhaust the list of relevant issues.

Medical historians have suggested that perhaps half of the first forty presidents of the United States suffered from some type of undiagnosed neuropsychiatric condition.[27] Both Abraham Lincoln and Franklin Pierce, for example, struggled with depression. Lyndon Johnson and Richard Nixon at times suffered from paranoia. Reagan in his later years was documented to suffer from dementia, diagnosed after he left office. President Woodrow Wilson had severe cognitive impairment because of a massive stroke that he suffered in office.

The American Psychiatric Association endorses what's referred to as the Goldwater Rule, which recommends that psychiatrists not diagnose any individuals with whom they have not had a face-to-face evaluation.[28] From an occupational medicine standpoint, in a job where the physical standards are codified—such as military service or special duty, like flight or a commercial driver's license, or if there is a codified fitness for duty involved in critical decision-making—then the neural cognitive function will be evaluated within stated critical decision-making guidelines.

The National Football League does cognitive ability testing on all potential players, most often using the Athletic Intelligence Quotient (AIQ), or S2 Cognition. No such requirement exists for our nation's leaders—and I wonder, why not?

For duties, offices, or positions unregulated by a written code—such as the president of the United States, a cabinet member, or a presidential appointee—then the neural cognitive function evaluation should follow critical decision-making guidelines and could be done as a baseline, taking into account anticipated occupational hazards for aging, or at the voluntary request of the individual. Basic critical decision-making guidelines say that the individual should have no mental, nervous, organic, or functional disease or psychiatric disorder likely to interfere with his or her ability to make critical decisions. Furthermore, a more detailed battery of tests should be administered rather than a screening test such as the MMSE or MoCA.

The second component is that the individual does not use a "controlled substance" identified in the Code of Federal Regulations, Title 21, Section 1308.11 Schedule 1, such as amphetamines, narcotics, or other habit-forming drugs. An obvious exception would be a substance or drug prescribed by a licensed medical practitioner familiar with the individual's personal history and occupation.

A third component is that the individual has no current clinical background of alcoholism.

Any evaluation would be conducted as a clinical examination, a neurological evaluation, and an assessment of neurophysiological and neuropsychological function. If there existed objective evidence of neurological dysfunction, then further investigation would be in order.

We don't routinely screen asymptomatic adults for cognitive impairment just because of their age. If cognitive difficulty is observed by a physician or if the family or patient has concerns about memory or cognition, then an evaluation to include screening is customary and the current standard of care. Medication and substance use history are evaluated, along with a depression screen. The physician should perform a complete physical exam including a neurological examination. A brief screening exam such as the MMSE or MoCA is indicated and useful. In addition to the usual battery of lab blood tests, B12 and thyroid function tests should be obtained. Genetic testing is not clinically correlated enough yet. An MRI and CT head scan are appropriate. This workup identifies most presumptive causes. A clinically active neurologist should be involved in the case. Specialized testing (lumbar puncture; brain biopsy; extensive, multi-day neuropsychological testing; and more advanced brain imaging) is only indicated for young presenting or rapidly progressing symptoms.

MOMENTOUS DECISIONS

All US presidents have exercised and will continue to exercise their choice of personal physician to provide healthcare while they remain in office. The president appoints the physician to the president, who serves as a White House commissioned officer in the Executive Office of the President, separate from the White House Military Office but supported by military medical personnel.

The assessment of "impairment" is a medical responsibility. The physician to the president, assisted by appropriate medical consultants, is responsible for determining and providing documentation of the full extent of how any impairment would affect the president's critical decision-making and executive functions. I don't think the physician to the president should routinely add mental screening tests to every physical. They should only be done when clinically indicated, with appropriate interpretation and follow-up. The physician to the president is also responsible for communicating and interpreting these findings, as needed, to the constitutionally designated decision-makers responsible for determining presidential "disability" (here meaning "inability" or "unable") under the provisions of the Twenty-Fifth Amendment.

The framers of the Twenty-Fifth Amendment clearly intended that decision-makers should solicit appropriate medical advice regarding the exercise of executive power under the amendment. Such momentous decisions should be made by accountable constitutional officials elected by the people, not by political commentators, the media, doctors, or attorneys.

PART THREE

—◆—

People, Pets, and Places
with the Presidents

12

POPES, QUEENS, AND EMPERORS

The history of civilization is written with the lives of conquerors, monarchs, emperors, and popes. As modern medicine has evolved, those rendering care to these leaders sometimes become a footnote in history.

Consider James Reid, a Scotsman physician who met Queen Victoria in 1881 at her Balmoral royal estate. He became her personal physician and close confidant, caring for her and her extended family for the rest of her life, and then for her successors, from Edward VII into the first years of the reign of George V.

While I never took care of a queen, emperor, or pope, I did get to meet some of them as a White House physician. And while I never made a visit to the Balmoral royal estate, I did get to stay briefly at Buckingham Palace—which is maybe worth a little tale of its own.

QUEEN ELIZABETH II

The United States and the United Kingdom have a special relationship going back to the founding of our country. Queen Elizabeth II (1926–2022) was the longest reigning monarch in history, spending sixty-three years on the throne over a period of fourteen US presidents.

The queen visited the United States several times, with official state visits to see President Dwight D. Eisenhower in 1957; President Gerald Ford in 1976 (to help commemorate the nation's bicentennial); and President George H. W. Bush in 1991, when she planted a tree on the South Lawn of the White House.. She also visited President Ronald Reagan at the Western White House in California in 1983, and in 2007 visited President George W. Bush to celebrate the four hundredth anniversary of the founding of Jamestown. History tells us why she might have chosen to attend the latter event.

On May 13, 1607, 104 men and boys on three English ships—the *Susan Constant*, the *Godspeed*, and the *Discovery*—picked the Jamestown site to build the first permanent English settlement in North America. At the time, Jamestown was surrounded by water on three sides and yet remained far inland, a defensible position against possible Spanish attack. Although the settlers finished their triangle-shaped fort on June 13, its walls could not keep out disease, hardship, and death. Many died from drinking salty or slimy water, and some estimates claim that 80–90 percent of the original settlers died in the first few years.

How would I have fared, I wonder, if I had arrived with them as the physician to the settlement? With modern medicine, pharmaceuticals, knowledge, and technology, I surely could have helped save many of those lives. But given the state of medicine at the time, would I have made much of a difference? Or would I have become one of the early casualties? We'll never know, and I suppose that's just as well.

The Virginia Company that founded Jamestown named the settlement after the English king, James I (1566–1625). Queen Elizabeth II was related to James I even though the House of Tudor had ended with the death of "the Virgin Queen," Queen Elizabeth I (1533–1603). Her royal family connection came through King Henry VIII's sister, Queen Margaret of Scotland, the grandmother of Mary, Queen of Scots. James I was the son of Mary, Queen of Scots.

Queen Elizabeth II came to the US for a state visit in May 2007 during a six-day royal tour. She first traveled to the Tidewater area of Virginia to mark the four-hundredth anniversary of Jamestown. She then spent a couple of days in Louisville, Kentucky. Most "queen watchers" believe the highlight of her trip came at the Kentucky Derby, as the queen was well known to be a horse racing/breeding aficionado. In fact, some say it was her personal passion and expertise.

On May 7, she arrived at the White House for a South Lawn arrival ceremony. Officially, the guest list contained seven thousand names. I was present and helped oversee the medical coverage for all those attending on the South Lawn. I had never seen that many people all congregating in that space. While seven thousand attendees may not seem huge, the actual attendance was almost certainly closer to nineteen thousand individuals.

In my sixteen years of association with the White House, it's the *only* event that my wife, Sandy, wanted to attend. With full official approval, she came to the White House and was among the throng of attendees on the South Lawn.

The royal motorcade pulled up, with appropriate greetings from President Bush and the First Lady to Queen Elizabeth II and the Duke of Edinburgh. Then the president of the United States and the sovereign of the United Kingdom went together to the reviewing platform. A twenty-one-gun salute welcomed them, and the national anthems of the United Kingdom and the United States were played. A decade and a half later, I can almost still hear "God Save the Queen" and "The Star-Spangled Banner" ringing out over the South Lawn of the White House.

After reviewing the troops, the two heads of state both made remarks and then moved to the Blue Room balcony on the state floor for photos.

Later that evening, the president hosted a state dinner, the only one I can remember that was white tie. The executive chef, Cris Comerford, had worked at the White House since 1995 but had become the executive chef two years before the queen's visit. A new executive pastry chef, Bill Yosses, started in January of 2007. I was privileged to provide medical advice and interact with both of those individuals when they needed it. Members of the WHMU don't make the guest list or fill a seat, but we are staffed up and located nearby to provide prompt medical care as needed.

Four years later, in May 2011, I got to visit Buckingham Palace while traveling with President Obama on his second trip to the UK. The First Lady referred to the visit as a "sleepover." Our hosts assigned me to quarters known as the Lord Chamberlain bedroom, a historic space outfitted with basic furniture. I remember the food provided: a plate of fruit with bananas, grapes, pears, and oranges. I also had been given two glass bottles of water, one still and one sparkling, each displaying the Royal Standard.

The next morning, we got up early and by 8:00 a.m. had departed from the lawn of Buckingham Palace in Marine One. We had two VH-3s in our flotilla, along with a couple of Phrogs (CH-46s, the workhorses of Marine Corps aviation for fifty years until they were phased out in 2015). We had the best aerial tour of London ever as we proceeded up the River Thames, taking in the sights on a gorgeous late spring morning.

Only two heads of state besides the president have ever been authorized to use the Marine One "White Top" helicopters during a visit to the United States. One was the queen. The other was the pope, whose story comes next.

POPE BENEDICT XVI

In April 2008, Pope Benedict XVI made his first visit to the United States in his official role as the bishop of Rome. It was only the second time a pope had visited the White House; Pope Paul VI was the first to visit in October 1965, more than four decades previously.

Pope Benedict's aircraft landed at Andrews Air Force Base. The papal motorcade, surrounded by Secret Service, slowly took him to the White House. There he was formally received with a South Lawn arrival ceremony.

Like the visit by the queen a year before, more than nineteen thousand individuals attended the event. I'd seen many large crowds at the White House, but I never saw more people crowd the South Lawn than for the two visits of the queen and the pope, probably because America is full of Anglophiles and Catholics.

Pope Benedict grew up as a Bavarian boy named Joseph Ratzinger; he was just six years old when the Nazis took power in Germany. He entered seminary in 1939 but two years later was forced to join the Hitler Youth. The German military drafted him into service in 1943 but he deserted within two years and was captured by American forces in 1945. He was ordained a priest in 1951, earned his doctorate in theology in 1953, and began a long academic career of teaching in several German universities. For more than two decades, he served as Pope John Paul II's closest advisor. He was elected pope on April 19, 2005, at age seventy-eight, making him the oldest pope to be elected since Clement XII (1652–1740). He served as pope from 2005 until his resignation in 2013, when he cited his age and health as reasons for his retirement. He thus became the first pope to resign since Gregory XII in 1415. The pope emeritus lived another nine years until his death in 2022.

I was the physician working in the doctor's office that day when Pope Benedict visited President Bush at the White House. I watched him up on the balcony overlooking the South Lawn, where those in attendance sang "Happy Birthday" to him. After the arrival ceremony, President Bush and Pope Benedict went inside, where a birthday cake waited for the pope, who was celebrating his eighty-first birthday.

I heard the president, the pope, and the group accompanying them as they all came down from the state floor; the layout of the Executive Mansion dictates that you must walk past the doctor's office on the ground floor. As President Bush reached our office, he stopped and motioned for the White House nurse, Cindy Wright, and me to come out. He first introduced Cindy to the pope. As a devout Catholic, she'd made it clear that she considered the experience one of the highlights of her life.

Earlier in the day, I had heard on NPR that anyone introduced to the pope could address him either as Holy Father or His Excellency, as he was the sovereign of his nation, the Holy See. The sovereign nation of Vatican City, situated completely inside the city of Rome, has the smallest population of any nation on earth (currently 764). During my introduction to the pope, I shook his hand and said, "Welcome, Your Excellency. Thank you for coming. I hope you have a productive visit." The White House photographer, Eric Draper, captured the moment in a photo. To this day, my kids' friends will look at the picture and ask, "Hey, who are those two old men with your dad? They look familiar."

The pope and the president then walked toward the West Colonnade by the Rose Garden. As they strolled away, I could hear Pope Benedict say to the president, in an astonished tone, "You allow non-believers to work here?"

The president kind of chuckled and replied, "We allow all faiths to work here."

President Bush knew that I was a protestant Christian and that therefore I didn't believe that any human is the Vicar of Christ on earth, one of the pope's many titles. The titles "pope" and "pontiff" both hail from about the mid–third century A.D., while most of the others originate somewhere between the fifth century and the Middle Ages. Americans use many titles to refer to the US president—commander in chief, head of state, POTUS, chief executive, chief diplomat, chief of party—but the president can't really compete with the pope, who is known variously as the Bishop of Rome, Vicar of Jesus Christ, Successor of the Prince of the Apostles, Supreme Pontiff of the Universal Church, Primate of Italy, Metropolitan Archbishop of the Roman Province, Sovereign of the Vatican City State, and Servant of the Servants of God. I suppose any office that continues for millennia probably deserves an abundance of titles.

I still remember the unique red shoes that the pope wore that day, the friendly demeanor that he exhibited, and that he spoke better English than I did. As I returned to my office, he and the president jovially chatted as they continued together past the Rose Garden to the West Wing and an Oval Office visit.

On that same visit, Pope Benedict later held a mass at the Washington Nationals' baseball stadium and then traveled up to New York City, where he addressed the UN General Assembly. He also held another mass at Yankee Stadium and visited the site of the former World Trade Center, where he prayed at Ground Zero to commemorate those killed in the terrorist attacks seven years earlier on 9/11.

One year later, I accompanied President Obama on a July 2009 visit to Vatican City, the most diminutive nation in the world at about 121 acres. That's about half of a square kilometer, or 120 times smaller than the island of Manhattan. We walked through several famous sites, including the Sistine Chapel in the Apostolic Palace, the pope's official residence. Officials there had cleared the place of tourists to accommodate the presidential visit, so our time there felt extra special.

EMPEROR AKIHITO

During President Obama's first year in office, we traveled to the annual APEC Summit, that year hosted in Singapore. We stopped in Tokyo, Japan, on November 13–14, 2009. During that visit, President Obama and a few senior staff visited the Imperial Palace, consisting of nearly half a square mile of historic buildings, including various residential and administrative palaces.

We pulled up to the main palace in the presidential motorcade. The president got out of the Beast (the president's armored limousine) and walked toward the entrance. The main palace had suffered significant damage in May 1945 during World War II due to Allied bombings, but within a couple of decades, it had been fully restored. Emperor Akihito greeted the president, who addressed him appropriately as "His Majesty." Out of state courtesy and following the cultural custom in Japan, President Obama gave the emperor a bow. The president's lanky body made his movement appear as an exaggerated, long movement, as captured by White House photographer Pete Sousa.

Only two individuals went in with President Obama for his private dinner with Emperor Akihito: the Marine Corps military aide and me. That was unique. We were led to another room while President Obama and the emperor had dinner alone.

I remember the irony at the time, thinking that the military aide who carried the nuclear codes had on his person the trigger that could unleash enough firepower to cause massive global death, destroy world peace, and disrupt the planetary order. That explains why some occasionally called him "Dr. Death." At the same time, there I was, the person who carries lifesaving equipment, which explains why some refer to the physician to the president as "Dr. Life." On that day, both Dr. Death and Dr. Life visited the only country on earth where nuclear weapons had been unleashed in wartime.

His Majesty, Emperor Akihito, was born at the Tokyo Imperial Palace in 1933. He was the oldest son of Emperor Hirohito, who ruled his nation for sixty-two years, the longest-reigning monarch in Japan's history. In 1989, when Emperor Hirohito died, Emperor Akihito ascended to the Chrysanthemum Throne. Some thirty years before, he had married a commoner named Michiko Shōda, shocking many traditionalists—no emperor before had ever married someone outside of the aristocracy.

Emperor Hirohito had been very involved with the hostilities of World War II. History reports him as landing on both sides of the controversy. The first time that his countrymen ever heard his voice was on August 15, 1945, when on radio he announced the unconditional surrender of his country. He told his people, "The enemy has begun to employ a new and most cruel bomb, the power of which to do damage is indeed incalculable, taking the toll of many innocent lives. Should we continue to fight, not only would it result in an ultimate collapse and obliteration of the Japanese nation, but it would also lead to the total extinction of human civilization."

Thirty years later, in 1975 (about fourteen years before his death), the emperor gave a press conference. When reporters asked him about the bombing of Hiroshima and Nagasaki, he replied, "It's very regrettable that nuclear bombs were dropped, and I feel sorry for the citizens of Hiroshima, but it couldn't be helped because that happened in wartime."

Personally, I consider the horrors that led up to the end of World War II—the only time in history that atomic weapons have been used—as nothing but tragedies. People today still debate President Truman's decision to use nuclear weapons, but the truth remains that the United States is the only nation on earth to detonate such a fearsome weapon over the cities of its enemy. And yet, a generation or two later, the United States and Japan have become the closest of allies. I witnessed that in person when the son of the emperor who ruled Japan during World War II sat down with the president of the United States to share a heartfelt meal. How I wish that could become the accepted norm.

HOLIDAYS AT THE WHITE HOUSE

While I enjoyed meeting queens, popes, and emperors (or at least stepping foot in their homes), I never grew tired of spending time with presidents and their families, especially during the holiday season. Christmas, in particular, was always a big occasion at the White House.

Staff shut down the Executive Mansion for tours just before Thanksgiving and kept it closed the entire week after Thanksgiving as they set up and decorated the house for the Christmas holiday. White House employees don't merely pull out boxes full of ornaments from the attic and put those on display. No, decorators take a full year to design each year's look, with new displays and arrangements and trimmings that they hope will thrill, inspire, and even awe visitors during that special, festive season.

President Bush was always very generous with his time, along with the First Lady, and they typically invited friends, family, and staff for one of the many White House parties that took place during the holidays. As a physician who worked with the medical unit, I attended with my colleagues on the last night of the holiday parties, known as "staff night."

Our four kids did not always appreciate the special privilege of experiencing an evening at a White House Christmas party. They knew only that they had to dress up and drive downtown during a busy time at the end of a school year, and that none of their classmates would be there. My eldest son, Michael, was a bit fussy at age nine. The First Lady, noticing his unhappiness, asked him what was wrong.

"There is nothing to eat here," he replied.

Apparently, the lavish holiday spread, exquisitely prepared and displayed, did not deliver whatever he was hoping for. We made sure on the drive home to stop and acquire a more pleasing food option for him.

On a happier note, I remember the First Daughters engaging with my young daughters. They commented on their names—Isabella and Selena—and told them both names were on their favorites list.

The Obamas were just as generous as the Bushes with their precious time during the holidays. Over the years, my whole family learned to look forward to the annual Christmas Party in the People's House.

Yes, even Michael.

13

PRESIDENTIAL PETS (AND POLITICAL PARTIES)

A relatively new phenomenon sweeping the country prompts some people to celebrate and others to cringe. You probably have seen a bumper sticker or two that simultaneously illustrates the current sensation and triggers debate.

"Fur baby on board," some of these bumper stickers say. "Dog Parent," announce others, or "Proud Pet Parent," or something similar. The owners of such cars treat their pets essentially as their children. They might or might not have human sons or daughters, but they consider their beloved dog, cat, or some other pet their human child.

Psychology Today noticed this trend a few years ago and in response published an article titled "Why Some People Think of Pets Like Children and Others Don't."[29] Author Vinita Mehta reported the results of a 2018 study by Nicole Owens and Liz Grauerholz, writing, "Welcome to the 21st century and interspecies families."

I must report that as a father and a family doctor, people often ask me for medical opinions about their pets or about the care of a beloved dog or cat belonging to family or friends. I assume they believe that learning about the anatomy, physiology, and pathophysiology of humans somehow extends to other species, specifically to domesticated mammals or rodents in the animal world.

And, in fact, some duties that fall to the physician to the president do indeed include taking care of a First Family's loved ones—and sometimes that includes their pets. While I don't know that I've ever heard a president or First Lady refer to a family pet as a "fur baby" or identify themselves as "proud pet parents," the reality is that presidential pets can receive and have received at least some type of care from the physician to the president.

And I am no exception.

PRESIDENTIAL DOGS

A frustrated President Harry S. Truman supposedly said, "if you want a friend in Washington, get a dog." It's up for debate whether he really uttered those words, but we do know that President Truman had two dogs.

After President Franklin Delano Roosevelt died on April 12, 1945, Vice President Truman became the new commander in chief. About two years later, a supporter from Missouri sent President Truman a cocker spaniel puppy named Feller. Feller became the Truman family's first dog.

I wonder if Feller, arriving at the White House as a puppy in December 1947, might have been named after Bob Feller, the flame-throwing pitcher for the Cleveland Indians of Major League Baseball. Bob Feller had taken a three-year break from professional baseball to serve his country during World War II, joining the US Navy.

At this point, I should back up a bit in this story to make clear the physician-pet connection. From mid-July to early August 1945, President Truman attended the Potsdam Conference, where he met with Joseph Stalin and Winston Churchill (and beginning on July 26, with Clement Attlee, who defeated Churchill in a July election). The leaders discussed Germany's surrender and tried to forge a path for peace and lay out a workable postwar world order.

President Truman's military aide, Brigadier General Harvey Vaughn, knew of a physician named Wallace Graham. The doctor had served in the army as a physician, even storming Omaha Beach in Normandy with the D-Day invasions. Dr. Graham had received his medical training at Creighton University in Omaha and went on to become a general surgeon. General Vaughn summoned Dr. Graham to meet the president, and after some discussions, President Truman offered Dr. Graham the job of White House physician.

In subsequent conversations, the pair discovered that President Truman knew Dr. Graham's father, a well-known physician in Kansas City. At that point, Dr. Graham accepted the job, moved to Washington D.C., and continued practicing surgery at the Walter Reed General Hospital while also serving as the physician to the president.

And now, back to the dog. Although Feller was an adorable cocker spaniel, it turned out that the Trumans weren't really dog people. President Truman therefore gave his pet canine to Dr. Graham, who, like Truman, was from Missouri. President Truman was widely known to be healthy, which meant that Dr. Graham didn't have to worry much about his primary patient's medical condition. No doubt that left the good doctor with a great deal of time to spend with Feller, his cocker spaniel gifted from the president.

President Truman is not the only president with a dog—or even the only one with a famous dog. According to some, President Herbert Hoover's Belgian Shepherd, King Tut, helped him win an election after the dog appeared in a campaign photo.

There have been post-revolutionary dogs, Civil War–era dogs, and Cold War dogs. Of the past forty-six US presidents, thirty-one of them kept at least one dog at 1600 Pennsylvania Avenue. Some pet always lived with the First Family between the presidencies of Andrew Jackson in the 1860s and Donald Trump (who had no pets), a stretch of 150 years.

The last pet to die at the White House was Champ, a German shepherd who joined the Biden family when Joe Biden became vice president. The dog got his name as a tribute to President Biden's father, who encouraged his son during difficult times by saying, "Get up, champ." When Champ died on June 19, 2021, the Biden family released a statement that said, "In our most joyful moments and in our most grief-stricken days, [Champ] was there with us, sensitive to our every unspoken feeling and emotion. We love our sweet, good boy and will miss him always."

BEYOND DOGS AND CATS

What kind of pets have lived in the White House? Dogs and cats, certainly, but they have had lots of company. A partial list of presidential pets includes hamsters, canaries, ponies, parakeets, a mockingbird, ducks, a squirrel, sheep, cows, a garter snake, a rooster, a badger, a goat, a fawn, horses, and bald eagles.

President Abraham Lincoln famously "pardoned" his pet turkey, Jack, one Thanksgiving Day. Sadly, President Lincoln's yellow Lab mix, Fido, was knifed by a drunken man after the president's own assassination.

The daughter of President Kennedy, Caroline, kept a pony at Camp David. She had "called it Macaroni," which, of course, echoes the famous song "Yankee Doodle Dandy." The Kennedy family had other horses, too. The First Lady had two of them, a piebald gelding named Rufus and an Arabian named Sardar. Caroline had a second horse named Tex, a Yucatan bay pony, given to her by Vice President Lyndon B. Johnson. John Jr. had Leprechaun, a Connemara pony given to the family by the people of Ireland. As the US's first Irish-Catholic president, John Fitzgerald Kennedy had a special connection to Ireland. All four of the president's grandparents were children of Irish immigrants, and he traced his Irish roots through both the Fitzgerald and Kennedy families.

The Kennedy pets didn't end there, either. Caroline was nearly three years old when her father was elected president, and John Jr. was born just days after the election. The Kennedys accumulated quite a menagerie of pets over their brief time in the White House:

two hamsters (Debbie and Billie), one cat (Tom Kitten), one canary (Robin), two parakeets (Bluebell and Maybelle), a Welsh terrier (Charlie), an Irish wolfhound (Wolf), a German shepherd (Clipper), a cocker spaniel (Shannon), a standard poodle (Gaullie), a mixed-breed dog (Pushinka) given to them by Soviet premier Nikita Khrushchev, and a rabbit (Zsa Zsa).

With all that presidential pet history, I suppose it's no surprise that I also entered a bit into that story.

A MARINE ONE BUDDY AND SOME SCOTTIES

My own interaction with presidential pets began in 2001, starting with Spot, an elderly English springer spaniel. As I've noted, President Bush liked to give everybody a nickname, including his dogs. That's how Spot soon became Spotty.

Spotty was the only presidential pet to serve in multiple administrations. She was born in 1989 at the White House to Millie, the pet dog of President George H. W. Bush. She died in the White House in 2004 at the ripe old age of fourteen.

Sometimes Spot would ride with me in the back of Marine One when I served as the on-duty physician. I always made sure that Spot got to sit in her preferred seat on the helicopter. When Spot made the short trip to Camp David, I took care that she always got off the helo safely and arrived wherever she needed to be.

President Bush spent much more time with his Scottie dogs than with Spotty. Barney was his first Scottie dog and quickly became the president's frequent companion at Prairie Chapel Ranch. Barney often rode around in a pickup truck with President Bush or joined him as he fished on the lake. Barney was a true companion, nearly a son, and was unfailingly supportive of the president's endeavors. A little later, a second Scottie dog came along, this one named Miss Beazley.

Whenever it became clear that Barney or Miss Beazley needed a medical evaluation or required some procedure, I felt useful by giving a quick opinion or coordinating their care with veterinarians in private practice. Sometimes the vets had offices in the area and at other times they worked at the army veterinary clinic in Fort Belvoir, Virginia.

The Bush twins, Jenna and Barbara, had a cat named India, but once more, President Bush felt compelled to give the beloved animal a nickname. And so, India became Willie, possibly named after the president's favorite baseball player, Willie Mays. I believe it had been President Bush's childhood ambition to grow up and be Willie Mays. While he fell far short of that lofty goal, at least he became president.

ALLERGIES AND PETS

When President Obama came into office in January 2009, it was public knowledge that his daughters suffered from allergies, specifically to pets. Obama nevertheless had made a campaign promise to Malia and Sasha that if he became president, he would get a family dog on inauguration day.

From the time the outgoing president leaves the White House until the incoming president arrives, there exists a several hour window of opportunity when the White House staff completely transforms everything in the presidential home to accommodate the new family. The process may include touch-up painting, fixing nicks or holes, or replacing any carpets that need to go.

As usual, the efficient and amazingly capable White House staff quickly turned over the entire residence, making sure that any cat or dog allergens from Barney, Miss Beazley, or India had been scrubbed clean from the house. By the time the Obama family moved in, no allergens remained. The Obamas had an allergy-free zone to live in on the second floor.

Senator Ted Kennedy, a close friend and colleague of President Obama, soon gifted a Portuguese water dog to the Obama family, which they named Bo. Bo was not very allergenic and a nice dog to have around; he often spent time both with the president and with other members of the family. He also liked to hobnob with various non-family members who worked in or frequented the White House.

As you might have guessed, sometimes that included those of us working in the WHMU. Bo liked to saunter into the doctor's office and make himself at home on the floor, or at other times on the couch (if he wanted more comfort). Many children of family or friends who visited me at the White House stated the highlight of their trip was meeting Bo.

SUPERSTAR GARDENER AND PET WHISPERER

Dale Haney is a true stalwart at making sure the White House is what it is. During my tenure there, I implicitly trusted Dale's advice and guidance. I quickly discovered that everyone else on the Eighteen Acres did so, too.

Dale is a superstar gardener and the superintendent of the White House grounds. In one quiet moment, Dale told me that he started in 1972 and that he was there on the dark day of August 9, 1974, when President Richard M. Nixon walked out of the White House for the last time. The president had just resigned his office—the only person ever to do so—strode across the South Lawn, boarded Marine One, waved to the crowd, and flew off into history.

Dale celebrated his golden work anniversary at the White House in 2022, which meant that he'd amassed more than fifty years of service to ten different presidents. When he arrived, he had intended to stay only two years; he wanted to return to school to add some academic heft to his bachelor's degree in horticulture.[30] He began his career on the Eighteen Acres as a foreman, then became the chief horticulturalist, and finally was promoted in 2008 to grounds superintendent. He reports to the chief usher and supervises a staff of twelve full-time employees.

Dale is the driving force behind what makes the Rose Garden and the First Lady's Garden (sometimes called the Jacqueline Kennedy Garden) spectacular. The Easter egg rolls, the state arrival ceremonies, the holidays (including Christmas), weddings—*everything* about the grounds looks impeccable 365 days a year. Dale is responsible for overseeing the care of hundreds of trees, thousands of shrubs, and most anything else that grows on the White House grounds.

Dale's ground floor office was in reasonable proximity to the doctor's office, situated close to the tradesmen's entrance. He spent most of his time in the gardens working, but on occasion, when he labored in his office trying to coordinate various White House events, he often found a happy friend eager to see him.

Bo, the Obamas' Portuguese water dog, *loved* to spend time with Dale, especially when Bo's presidential parents were off elsewhere doing the people's work. Dale always made sure that Bo was well taken care of.

And Bo wasn't Dale's first furry White House friend, either—not by a long shot. Some know Dale best by his unofficial title as "the keeper of the president's pets."

"The first thing I think about when I think about Dale is his relationship with the First Family's animals," said Gary Walters, who for more than twenty years served as the White House chief usher.[31] "He's like the whisperer," added Anita McBride, who worked as an aide in President Reagan's correspondence office and later returned to work for the administrations of both Bush 41 and Bush 43.[32]

Dale has taken great pleasure in walking many presidential dogs, from Richard Nixon's Irish setter, King Timahoe, to Joe Biden's German shepherd, Commander. During 9/11, when nearly all of us had evacuated the White House, Dale was spotted still standing on the South Lawn, holding Barney under one arm and Willie under the other. Both pets were later reunited with First Lady Laura Bush at a remote location. Mrs. Bush called Dale "the best friend of all the animals" and declared that "our dogs Spot, Barney, and Beazley adored him. They loved him more than they loved us."[33]

MORE THAN DONKEYS AND ELEPHANTS?

As I think about presidential pets over the centuries, I wonder if our nation might be better off if it took a page out of White House history and adopted more than the two national pets we currently have. Donkeys and elephants are great, but why limit ourselves to them?

I think back to our Founding Fathers, who warned us against getting too comfy with any particular political party. Not until our eighth president, Martin Van Buren, "Old Kinderhook," did we get cozy with just two major parties. Back then, it was the Jacksonian Democrats and the Whigs. Today, it's the Democrats and the Republicans.

The financial crisis of 1837 dogged Van Buren's presidency and made him into a political pariah, but he seems to me to have been a decent man who lived a respectable life, despite having an unremarkable presidency. I like what historian Mark Cheathem has written about him:

> If Van Buren were alive today, I think he would tell us all that we have forgotten political parties are, at their heart, made up of the people, and that it is the job of the people to bring the parties back into harmony with constitutional principles that benefit the good of the whole nation rather than special interests that divide us.[34]

Today, unfortunately, our two major political parties have a stranglehold on political leadership in the US and seem to do whatever it takes to stay in power. It's often been said that the American electorate gets the leader they choose . . . and deserve.

I also think of an old story that asks, "Would you rather give someone a fish or teach them how to fish?" Personally, I'd rather teach them how to fish, but I'd also want to make sure that some fish are swimming in the lake where they're fishing.

Finally, I'd say that if our donkeys and elephants can't figure out how to work together to make this work, then maybe, just maybe, we should start looking for some additional pets.

A President's Best Friend

Dogs can form deep bonds with humans. Dogs rely on their humans for a sense of security, safety, affection, and comfort. In a most demanding environment, such as the White House or inside the presidential bubble, interaction and relationship with beloved pets helps remind the president and First Family of their humanity.

It is priceless to have a friend who accepts you unconditionally and asks for nothing in return other than to love and be loved. Dogs and other pets support human health and well-being. They, too, can be a part of whole person care. Maybe one sound piece of medical advice from doctor to patient should be this: get a dog and spend some time together.

14

WHEN PRESIDENTS VISIT WAR ZONES

US presidents have a long history of visiting active war zones, beginning at least with Abraham Lincoln. After Confederate forces under Lieutenant General Jubal Early attacked Fort Stevens on July 11, 1864, President Lincoln left the Executive Mansion the next day to visit the battlefield. He didn't have to go far—the Union fort stood less than four miles from the White House.

The story goes that when the president climbed a parapet at the fort to get a better view of the skirmish, enemy troops started firing at him. A Union soldier is said to have shouted at the commander in chief, "Get down, you damned fool!" While President Lincoln escaped the incident unharmed, a Union surgeon standing just a few feet from him was hit and wounded. Confederate troops withdrew from the area after two days of light action.

Less than a year later, on April 4, 1865, President Lincoln visited Richmond, Virginia, just two days after Confederate forces abandoned the former capital of the South. Secretary of War Edwin Stanton did not think much of the visit, writing in a telegram to the president,

"Allow me respectfully to ask you to consider whether you ought to expose the nation to the consequences of any disaster to yourself in the pursuit of a treacherous and dangerous enemy like the rebel army."

President Lincoln responded, "I will take care of myself."[35]

He nearly had to. As the president and his son, Tad, attempted to reach and tour the former Confederate White House—by then transformed into the US military's headquarters—"only a few sailors were on hand to guard the President against attack . . . Military authorities eventually spotted the President and guided him to the house once occupied by Jefferson Davis, President of the Confederacy."[36]

President Lincoln and Tad spent that night aboard the USS *Malvern*, a Union warship docked at Rocketts Landing. General Robert E. Lee surrendered four days later, and less than a week after that, Southern sympathizer John Wilkes Booth shot the president in the head as he watched *Our American Cousin* at Ford's Theatre in Washington, D.C. President Lincoln died on April 15, 1865.

MODERN VISITS TO WAR ZONES

In modern times, US presidents have frequented war zones more often and with more security than in the past. During World War II, President Franklin Delano Roosevelt visited Casablanca in January 1943 as Allied forces assaulted Tripoli. He visited military installations in Italy on December 8, 1943, traveling in a jeep with Allied Supreme Commander Dwight D. Eisenhower (and with General George S. Patton tagging along behind). He participated in the Malta Conference with Britain's prime minister Winston Churchill in February 1945. That same month, he met with both Churchill and the Soviet premier, Joseph Stalin, at the Yalta Conference to discuss the reorganization of Germany and Europe after the end of the war.

The president did all this while dealing with a physical impairment resulting from what is generally thought to have been a battle with polio.[37] Since then:

- President-Elect Dwight D. Eisenhower visited Korea on November 29, 1952, fulfilling a campaign promise to go there to try to find a way to end the conflict, which had raged since 1950. An armistice was signed during his presidency on July 27, 1953.
- President Lyndon Baines Johnson took two trips to Cam Ranh Bay in Vietnam, the first in October 1966 and the other in December 1967. He had first ordered troops to Vietnam in March 1965.
- President Richard M. Nixon took one trip to Vietnam, on July 30, 1969, when he met with South Vietnamese president Nguyen Van Thieu and visited US troops stationed in Saigon.
- President Ronald Reagan made a stop for lunch in South Korea at Camp Liberty Bell in the DMZ in November 1983.
- President George H. W. Bush made a surprise Thanksgiving Day stop on November 22, 1990, to visit US troops massed in the Saudi Arabian desert—and to serve them Thanksgiving dinner—during Operation Desert Shield.
- President Bill Clinton made a July 1993 visit to US troops in the DMZ at Camp Casey in South Korea, and in January 1996 visited troops at Tuzla Air Base in Bosnia and Herzegovina.

In this chapter I'll focus on my involvement with a few war zone visits during service to Presidents Bush and Obama. Let's start with the ultimate crisis event for presidential military travel during my time at the White House.

THE WATERSHED EVENT: 9/11

Without question, 9/11 triggered a new round of presidential visits to war zones. Almost three thousand people died in the terrorist attacks of September 11, 2001, while thousands more were injured.

Within a month of the tragedy, President George W. Bush ordered the United States military to go on the attack against the Taliban in Afghanistan. The Taliban—members of a militant organization driven by a fundamentalist ideology that is part Pashtun nationalism and part self-professed Islamic purist—both assisted and encouraged the al-Qaeda terrorists who carried out the 9/11 attacks. The first US troops to be sent to Afghanistan were Special Forces units. In the fall of 2001, General Tommy Franks, who had taken command of the US Central Command in June 2000, led the American military efforts in Afghanistan.

In late December 2001, I was with the president at his Prairie Chapel Ranch during the holiday break. General Franks and his aide-de-camp flew directly from CENTCOM headquarters at MacDill Air Force Base in Tampa, Florida, into Central Texas, still wearing their desert fatigues. On December 28, they met face-to-face with the president to give him and his war council an up-to-date report on how the nation's military efforts were going in Afghanistan.

General Franks was no stranger to the Bush family even before he joined the military. He had attended Midland High School in Midland, Texas, along with First Lady Laura Bush, and although he belonged to the class one year ahead of her, they knew each other. So, as they shared a hamburger on the Prairie Chapel Ranch in late December, they had a lot to talk about and catch up on.

As the CENTCOM commander, General Franks had a lot to say. He reported how a tape of Osama bin Laden had surfaced. Speculation about bin Laden's whereabouts and a leaked report regarding the possibility of establishing tribunals provided timely topics. He also gave a frank assessment of the first few months of the nation's war efforts and provided some realistic perspectives of what lay ahead, especially in view of the challenging physical and cultural environment of Afghanistan.

President Bush experienced that challenging environment first-hand several years later. However, his first trip to a combat zone was when he visited troops stationed in Iraq during the Thanksgiving break of 2003.

Before the holiday break, the president had traveled to Prairie Chapel Ranch along with the First Lady, his parents, and extended family. During the dark of the night, the president slipped out for a clandestine trip overseas, accompanied by the Secret Service.

The presidential group flew from Texas back to Andrews Air Force Base outside of Washington, D.C., and changed planes in the hangar housing the presidential airlift group. The plane was filled with the usual Air Force One staff and passengers, as well as the traveling media pool, all of them sworn to secrecy. They flew directly to Baghdad International Airport on November 27, landing during the cover of night.

The American contingent remained on the ground for a few hours while President Bush met with the Coalition Provisional Authority and the Iraqi Governing Council. He also met with troops and military personnel stationed in Baghdad, delivering an encouraging speech to them at the Bob Hope Dining Facility.

After Air Force One took off and footage of the trip was released to the media, President Bush returned to Prairie Chapel Ranch and resumed the Thanksgiving holiday with his family, where I provided medical support during their time at the ranch.

President Bush took his first trip to Afghanistan on March 1, 2006, when he had an unannounced stop at Bagram Air Base in Kabul. There he met with Afghan president Hamid Karzai and dedicated the new US embassy. That trip took place while he was en route to India and Pakistan for scheduled visits.

In September 2007, I was on the Air Force One support plane trailing President Bush on Air Force One, headed to the Asia-Pacific Economic Cooperation Summit in Sydney. Instead of flying west, we flew east and stopped at Al-Asad Air Base in Iraq, where the president met with General David H. Petraeus, the secretary of state, the secretary of defense, and other senior officials, as well as with US troops. During that visit, Dr. Tubb, the physician to the president, followed the president around, which meant that I had the opportunity to visit the multinational forces hospital staffed by the 399th Combat Support Hospital (CSH). I wanted to see the outstanding medical care and facilities that had been prepared for our troops in that combat zone.

While there, I ran into Captain Frick, a senior naval flight surgeon whom I had known from previous duty stations. Wherever we looked on base, the thermometers read 111 degrees Fahrenheit. That's hot no matter where you're from. Seared into my memory is the presence and persistence of dust everywhere I looked. That dust permeated my clothing for weeks.

After the president and his staff had an uneventful visit in Iraq, we all continued around the world, stopping for an unannounced refueling at Diego Garcia, a strategic US military base in the Indian Ocean. We arrived bright and early at the crack of dawn, and at this small naval support facility—just a few square miles in size, built on a coral atoll and used by both the United States and the United Kingdom—I marveled at the view *and* at the temperature.

We had just left vast stretches of sand and 111-degree temperatures, and here the thermometer read a steady 80 degrees in the middle of the deep blue Indian Ocean. No official events had been planned in Diego Garcia; it was simply a routine fuel stop. We had been instructed not to wake the president, as we were en route to Sydney, Australia, for a summit.

But when President Bush looked out his window, he saw a formation of troops assembled at the naval support facility. "Absolutely," he said, "I'm going out there and paying tribute to the soldiers, sailors, and airmen who are deployed here protecting America."

When you're the president of the United States, plans have a way of changing quickly. He immediately left the plane and spent time with the troops as Air Force One refueled. We waited until he returned to the plane so we could continue our flight to the APEC Summit in Sydney.

THE WAR IN IRAQ

A year and three months later, General Franks led the initial US invasion of Iraq. That operation began in March 2003 and lasted about a month, resulting in the overthrow of Saddam Hussein on April 9.

US troops captured Hussein about eight months later, finding him hiding in an underground shelter. Three years later, in December 2006, Hussein was convicted. He was executed on December 30.

I was at Prairie Chapel Ranch on December 30, 2006, when, once more, President Bush received several briefings on world events, including the death of the dictator. About five years had elapsed between General Franks's Afghanistan briefing and the one regarding Saddam Hussein's execution. On both of those historic days, President Bush began his morning by running or cycling, followed by clearing brush after breakfast.

THE DMZ

The demilitarized zone separating North and South Korea is technically an active combat zone, more than seven decades after an armistice was signed. President Bush visited in February 2002. An iconic photo of President Bush shows him lifting a large pair of binoculars to his eyes after someone handed them to him. He immediately noticed the unremoved covers and took them off to have a look across the DMZ.

The president had arrived via Marine One from the army base in Seoul. In the cozy Blackhawk, I remember Secretary of State Colin Powell narrating, pointing out landmarks and the multiple bases where he had been stationed or where he'd commanded during his long and illustrious army career. The president and his entourage later ate lunch with servicemen stationed at the DMZ.

Observation posts, imposing barbed wire fences, and pre-positioned military equipment for miles around remind all who visit South Korea of the heightened state of alert required to be prepared for the unexpected.

PRESIDENT OBAMA IN IRAQ

In early April 2009, after President Obama had his first European swing attending G20, NATO, and US-EU summits, we made an unannounced visit to Iraq after a three-day visit to Turkey. In Baghdad, President Obama spoke and was warmly greeted at Camp Victory. Air Force major Ken Barron, who served as the advance officer and the tactical medical officer during President Obama's lone visit to Iraq, also served, for a time, as the senior physician assistant for the WHMU. In that capacity, Ken had provided on-site medical care during a February 2006 quail hunt in southern Texas with Vice President Dick Cheney.

The hunt unexpectedly made national headlines when the vice president accidentally shot a member of his hunting party with a 28-gauge shotgun. The victim, a seventy-eight-year-old Texas lawyer named Harry Whittington, was taken by ambulance to nearby Kingsville, then airlifted to Corpus Christi. He suffered a non-fatal heart attack a few days later, possibly because one or more lead-shot pellets from the vice president's shotgun had lodged near his heart. Mr. Whittington survived the incident and lived until February 2023.

Army captain Sarah Creason traveled with us on the Iraq trip as our critical care nurse. We visited an ornate Baghdad palace previously belonging to Saddam Hussein and noted that many US troops continued to be stationed there. The soldiers came out to see President Obama, greeting him as a rock star and a great celebration of American values and patriotism was on display.

BACK TO AFGHANISTAN AND IRAQ

President Obama focused the first few months of 2010 on Obamacare. On March 27, we did an over-and-back trip to Afghanistan, the president's first of three visits to that nation. We visited Kabul and Bagram Air Base, where he met with President Karzai. The president also met with a Navy SEAL team during that visit.

The advance officer for the WHMU on that trip was Commander Ronny Jackson, who also served as the tactical medical officer. The

Air Force One nurse who traveled with me was Navy lieutenant commander Chellie Carr.

Later that year, we returned to Bagram on December 3, where President Obama met with many military and diplomatic personnel to thank them for their hard work. On the flight home, I spent part of my time working with the president's valet on an injury he'd suffered while supporting the president. Of course, we utilized the medical unit on Air Force One.

On May 1, 2012, we flew back to Kabul. I remember that trip vividly because, once again, we landed hours after sunset. We all boarded helicopters and flew by the dark of night in blacked-out aircraft. President Obama met with President Karzai and signed a long-term strategic partnership. On that trip, the Air Force One nurse was Air Force major Susie Maroon, while the military aide was Major Reggie McClam. Pete Souza, White House photographer extraordinaire, managed to take excellent photos using only the available moonlight.

President Obama took one more trip to Afghanistan, in May 2014, after I retired from the navy.

THE MOST IMPORTANT THING

The most important thing about presidential flights, especially presidential visits to active combat zones, is the secrecy required. The "need to know" is kept to a bare minimum so that the enemy has no knowledge of the trip and therefore cannot assault the president or thwart the mission.

From a medical standpoint, we relied upon the medical care and trauma plans already in place for US military personnel. But we also had to know, confirm, and be able to blend into the existing travel plan as well as the overflight plan, which laid out the Level I trauma centers around the world that are part of the flight path of Air Force One.

Whenever we visited an active US combat zone, we fell into the plan of the Department of Defense, which had developed possibly the best trauma care in history for combatants. If it's good enough for our active-duty military, then it's absolutely good enough for the commander in chief.

One additional option for transportation, besides ground transport—we always set up a medivac option—was to use Marine One in case of any medical evacuation that needed to go from point A to a hospital landing zone. Teams also would rehearse or practice for Marine One in advance of the president's visit.

HE'S THERE AND HE CARES

Presidents routinely make decisions affecting the lives of millions, choices that can last for generations, even though each president remains on the world stage for only a short time. When leaders have that kind of massive authority and power, they need to show the people they lead that they care for them.

When the commander in chief visits a war zone, it's an opportunity not only to visit the newly wounded (who often still are in shell shock) but also a chance to learn firsthand the impact of some presidential decision. The visit enables these leaders to get an unvarnished assessment of how things are going, even in a hyper-controlled setting.

The president of the United States can't care if he's not there.

George W. Bush often said that after a natural disaster, such as a hurricane, tornado, or flood, leaders *must* show up to show their people that they care. The very same thing can be said about man-made disasters such as war.

You can't care if you're not there. Leaders *must* show up and let their people know that they care. And if that means visiting a war zone, despite the heightened dangers, they do it.

15

LET'S NOT MAKE TONIGHT'S NEWS

One of the challenges of serving as the physician to the president is providing comprehensive, professional healthcare to the president and all those who travel with him without putting your own work in the headlines. Your activity can't become a story, because that might seriously hinder and even jeopardize the agenda of the president.

I remember one medical advance team to Ulaanbaatar—the largest city in Mongolia and the coldest capital city in the world—who went out for a hike with some local embassy staff the day before a presidential visit. They took a wrong turn and spent the rest of the day and half the night unable to prepare for the big event. They were fortunate enough to stay alive. Luckily, they did not become the news.

While I was privileged to serve at the White House, I was personally involved with hundreds of medical scenarios that didn't make the headlines, some of them inside the US and many others overseas. Most of these incidents could be characterized as routine, although a few of them were anything but. In every case, though, the goal is always to provide the best medical care possible without drawing attention to what happened behind the scenes. A key part of the job of the physician to the president is to enable people to do their jobs without cameras getting in the way.

MEDICAL SUPPORT IN THE US

While emergency medical needs might seem to pop up more frequently while traveling overseas than while at home, the truth is that disease, accidents, and injuries of various kinds can and do intrude wherever human beings go. I offer the following abbreviated list of US cases merely to provide an idea of the ongoing day-in, day-out situations that require the attention of every physician to the president.

At the White House Medical Clinic
- Subarachnoid hemorrhage
- Appendicitis
- Cardiac arrest
- Stroke
- Insulin coma
- Self-immolation outside the White House gates
- A shooter who himself got shot and then fell outside the White House gate

At Prairie Chapel Ranch in Texas
- Injuries while using chainsaws requiring basic first aid
- Head injuries, whether lacerations from normal physical activities or falls from bicycles, including head and neck lacerations
- A fall causing a pneumothorax (Often called a "collapsed lung," it's caused when air gets into the chest outside of the lungs because of a fall or impact. Symptoms typically include chest pain, shortness of breath, tightness in the chest, and turning blue.)
- Five marines fell ill one summer day with heat stroke and hallucinations. We had prepared for the possibility and all five marines received prompt medical treatment, recovering with no lasting consequences.
- A child disappeared beneath a body of water on a nearby ranch. We summoned underwater rescue divers who

quickly found the four-year-old, who we then intubated. We called in a helicopter and evacuated the child to a hospital.

At Other Locations around the US

- Several cases of rash, later diagnosed as Lyme disease
- A hand fracture and gunshot wound to the face and chest, suffered on a hunting trip in South Texas
- A knee injury suffered by a school principal in South Florida
- Multiple cases of cardiac arrest and resuscitation at various sites in the United States. We provided initial care and then turned the patients over to local emergency medical services.

TRAVELING OVERSEAS

Over the past thirty years, the travel of US presidents to foreign countries has gone from a once-in-an-administration occurrence to a monthly, even routine event. With Air Force One at their beck and call, presidents can do a lot of work and yet rest and recover, all in the air, allowing them to make the most of their time at various summits or face-to-face meetings with world leaders.

Overseas travel regularly takes the presidents to austere places with very limited in-country medical resources. The physician to the president must come prepared to respond to whatever medical crisis may occur.

In my years with the White House Medical Unit, I've sewn up several individuals on Air Force One. Often, they had injured themselves carelessly, such as hitting their head on a helicopter. There's never a shortage of drama.

Countless medical cases requiring treatment occur while traveling abroad. To give you an idea, consider just a few typical instances:

- Triage care for multiple casualties after an explosion in Turkey
- Helped riders and multiple policemen injured on bicycles during a state visit to the United Kingdom, just before a state dinner

- Chest pain in the dark of the night on Air Force One over the Atlantic Ocean
- A bleed caused by a grenade explosion in the Republic of Georgia
- Multiple cases of viral labyrinthitis after a summit
- Several cases of dengue fever after traveling to San José, the capital of Costa Rica
- A fifty-year-old advance officer stricken with urosepsis and multi-organ failure
- A case of appendicitis, surgically repaired by a support team working in a Nigerian hotel room
- A case of dengue fever upon returning from Brazil
- More than 120 patients cared for during one visit to Cairo
- Altitude illness
- Cases of supraventricular tachycardia (PSVT, faster than normal heart rate) requiring evaluation
- Policemen suffering anaphylaxis (an allergic reaction that involves the whole body) in Cape Town, South Africa
- A twenty-six-year-old presented with a cough, shortness of breath, hypoxia, and sounds in the right hemithorax. He later received a chest tube and was evacuated to the National Institutes of Health, where he was diagnosed with a malignant pleural effusion.

Since we often visited nations located in malaria hot zones, ahead of the trip we researched the specific location, learned the local medical intelligence, and tried to ensure that our people got on proper malaria prophylaxis.

But not all individuals follow the protocols.

Three times I diagnosed malaria cases, once each upon our return from Benin, Ghana, and Nigeria. The first step in diagnosing malaria is to know the individual's recent travel history. Then you must communicate with the physician attending the patients to make sure they are being assessed accurately, receiving appropriate treatment, and getting the right lab work done.

Our goal was to provide medical care to those supporting the president and keep our patients out of the news, even under tricky international circumstances in, at times, resource-limited countries.

ENCEPHALITIS IN DUBAI

I served as the backup physician for a presidential trip to the Middle East in January 2008. I flew on the support plane, and as we landed in Abu Dhabi, United Arab Emirates, I received a call from our advance officer in Dubai. Lieutenant Commander Paul Klimkowski, an experienced navy physician's assistant, told me that a Secret Service member visiting a local coffee shop had suffered a grand mal seizure, the first such incident in his life.

"Take him to our trauma-designated hospital," I told him, "and ask for this doctor." Paul did so, and there the officer received an inpatient evaluation. We flew into Dubai for a day and then continued to Sharm el-Sheikh, Egypt. I called the attending doctors and suggested they start their patient on Acyclovir, an antiviral medication delivered intravenously. As they started to get the officer ready for an MRI, a technical problem with the equipment caused a delay. Once they fixed the problem and completed the MRI, they determined that our agent had herpes encephalitis, a brain infection with a 70 percent mortality rate.

The man stabilized after a few days, and through another phone conversation with his doctors, we determined that in another few days he should be ready for transport. I then coordinated a medivac to take him from Dubai to the encephalitis treatment unit at Johns Hopkins in Baltimore, Maryland.

He spent several weeks in recovery at Johns Hopkins, where his family could meet and support him. He was later moved to a longer-term rehab facility in Rochester, New York. Although he had to take an extended medical leave of absence from the Secret Service, he later worked in a support role.

It was an exciting day for me personally when about a year later he walked into my White House doctor's office and said, "I don't remember anything about that year of my life, but I understand you were involved with my care. I want to thank you." He still has some long-term issues, but he lived and is rehabilitating himself back to a normal life. This story demonstrates the importance of advance planning including the right hospitals and doctors to go to everywhere we went. It's a story that can be told countless times.

Nontyphoidal Salmonella Sepsis in Ghana

A thirty-year-old military communications officer working with the White House Communications Agency (WHCA) served as an advance officer in Accra, Ghana. After he had been in the country for a few days, he developed a rapid onset high fever, high heart rate, low blood pressure, disabling back pains, was hypoxic with respiratory distress, and became disoriented.

When I flew into Accra with my team, I evaluated him and arranged for a medivac on the Air Force One backup, on which I served as the medical officer. As we took off, I hooked him up to IVs, gave him antibiotics, and put him on oxygen.

After we landed eighteen hours later at Andrews Air Force Base in Prince George's County, Maryland, we took him to the intensive care unit at Walter Reed. He turned out to have nontyphoidal salmonella septic shock, which back then had about a 50 percent mortality rate. We figured that he ate some bad chicken, or something like it. He stayed a week or two in the ICU and recovered fully. Because of our advance planning, the team was able to provide him with extraordinary care, thereby saving his life.

Hand Injury in Dar es Salaam, Tanzania

We traveled in February 2008 with President Bush to Dar es Salaam, Tanzania. An Air Force One logistics staff member moving equipment around on the airport's tarmac sustained a serious hand injury right before Air Force One loaded up and moved on to Kigali, Rwanda.

I examined the airman, determined he had an open finger fracture, stabilized it on board Air Force One, and managed to call ahead to the Air Force Mobile Forward Surgical Team (MFST) team in Kigali that we had stationed at the US embassy just in case. The orthopedic surgeon and the nurse anesthetist there were able to pin the finger while the president attended an event. We then took the injured airman back home with us and turned over his care to hand surgeons in the United States.

BEIJING 2008: MORE THAN OLYMPIC EVENTS

I did the pre-advance for President Bush's visit to Beijing for the 2008 Summer Olympics, as I had for many pre-advances over the previous decade. One of the first meetings you typically have is with the local US embassy medical staff.

I met the State Department medical officer assigned to the embassy in Beijing and couldn't help but note his excitement about the approaching Olympics. He felt especially jazzed since he would be in the command center during the competition.

When he asked if I would like him to arrange a spot for me, I politely declined. The physician and the nurse on duty with the president travel around the city with him, I explained. They must always stay within two minutes of the president.

"And you can't provide care if you're not there," I said.

Earlier I had asked to see the most capable hospitals in Beijing, so the embassy physician scheduled a tour arranged by the Chinese government. The tour included a military hospital near "the Bird's Nest," the not-quite-finished Olympic site where construction crews were just finishing their work.

"Thank you for this," I said, "but I really would like to see Peking Union Medical College Hospital." I knew from prior visits that Peking

Union was the most capable trauma hospital in Beijing. The man reluctantly arranged a visit.

I also wanted to see a private hospital called the Beijing United Family Hospital, which I knew offered good cardiac care. We hoped to contract with that facility to make its ambulance part of our motorcade. But since Beijing Family wanted an exorbitant amount of money to provide the service (which seemed like highway robbery to the US government), we decided instead to bring along a US Secret Service ambulance.

One good thing happened during my visit to Beijing Family, however. I met Dr. Joe Passanante, a US-trained emergency medicine physician who spoke Mandarin and who knew well the capabilities of various hospitals in Beijing. Dr. Passanante was part of the group that had volunteered to help staff our emergency medical services crew.

During our visit to Peking Union, the staff very proudly showed us a new VIP ward—but think luxury, not medical capability. During the walkthrough, I asked to see where a trauma victim would come in. I also asked to view the emergency department entrance, a helicopter landing pad, possible decontamination facilities, and the resuscitation room. I was full of questions.

"How do you get to the operating room?" I asked. "How do you get to the intensive care unit? Do you bypass the typical post-anesthesia care unit?"

I very forcibly explained that we had to prepare for the unthinkable: a gunshot wound, a knife stabbing, somebody falling down some stairs and cracking open their head. How would we get them to definitive care? How could we give care under fire? How would we turn patients over to the trauma team?

Dozens of times, the Chinese security team emphatically repeated, "That will not happen here," or "That is not allowed," or "No gunshots, no knife attacks, no stabbings. This will never happen here." I had apparently offended them by insinuating that we should even *prepare* for a possible gunshot wound or knife stabbing, so I waited to ask my next question.

"If those things *did* happen," I asked, "where is the trauma team?"

The trauma team would be at home, they replied, and would be summoned to the hospital. They would make sure the team arrived in time to deliver the required care.

Very nicely and patiently, I explained that in the US or at international events like the Beijing Olympics, where travel is extremely controlled and extremely difficult, it always worked best if we had the trauma teams pre-positioned at the hospital.

They thought over my comments, agreed, and returned to me with an updated plan. They promised to have two teams ready to go. Team A would stay at the hospital for twenty-four hours, and then Team B would relieve them—an arrangement we found acceptable.

Opening Ceremony

The opening ceremony for the Beijing Olympics was held on August 8, 2008. Many Chinese consider the number eight both symbolic and lucky, associating it with being rich or well off.

We arrived in Beijing earlier that day with President Bush, his immediate family, Bush 41, and the extended Bush family. Our advance parties had arrived several days before. Secret Service personnel considered the logistics very challenging, as dozens of world leaders and heads of state were scheduled to attend the big event.

From an excerpt of *Decision Points*, authored by President George W. Bush in 2010:

> At the Opening Ceremony of the Olympics, Laura and I were seated in the same row as Vladimir [Putin] and his interpreter. This was the chance to have the conversation I had put off in the Great Hall. Laura and the man next to her, the king of Cambodia, shifted down a few seats. Putin slid in next to me. I knew the TV cameras would be on us, so I tried not to get overly animated. I told him he'd made a serious mistake, and

that Russia would isolate itself if it didn't get out of Georgia. He said Saakashvili was a war criminal—the same term Medvedev had used—who had provoked Russia.

"'I've been warning you Saakashvili is hot-blooded," I told Putin.

"I'm hot-blooded, too," Putin retorted.

I stared back at him. "No, Vladimir," I said. "You're cold-blooded."

The main part of the Georgian conflict lasted five days, from August 7 to 12, although shelling had begun between partisans on August 1. On August 12, Russia called a halt to the invasion and agreed to a six-point diplomatic push for peace led by France.

During the five-day conflict, 176 Georgian servicemen were killed, 14 policemen died, 228 civilians perished, and 1,747 were wounded. On the Russian side, 67 Russian soldiers were killed, 283 wounded, and 365 servicemen and civilians sympathetic to the Russians died, according to an EU fact-finding report.[38]

August 8 was not such a lucky day for any of *them*.

Crash and Suture

On the day after the opening ceremony, the president found himself with a two-hour window in his busy schedule. As per his custom, he'd also brought along his mountain bike. Three years before, he'd tried out Beijing's Laoshan Mountain Bike Course and he wanted to ride on it again. So, after an early wake-up call on Saturday, he took another scheduled ride on the Olympic course.

A military aide named Bob Roncska, an engineer and submarine officer in the US Navy, was off duty at the time. When on duty, "Navy Bob"—the president's nickname for him (and by the way, that nickname also stuck)—often carried the "nuclear football" for the president. On this morning, Navy Bob, a triathlete, went riding with President Bush, who cycled for about an hour. Somewhere on the course, Navy Bob went over an embankment, crashed, and opened a deep gash on his chin.

Dr. Joe Passanante, the physician I'd met earlier at Beijing Family, now riding as the ambulance medical attendant along with presidential nurse Cindy Wright, brought Navy Bob back to the St. Regis hotel where I was staying. I took the injured man to my hotel room and used my travel equipment to numb and clean him up. I assessed the wound, did vertical mattress sutures to close the extensive laceration on his chin, and put a nice dressing on it.

Throughout my work, Navy Bob expressed some concern about the result. "Do we need a plastic surgeon?" he wondered aloud. "Are you sure you know what you're doing?"

"You realize I have a needle and I'm sewing you up," I answered.

A few hours later, after I sent Navy Bob back to duty, President Bush himself expressed how very impressed he was with the top-notch care that Navy Bob had received. Sure, Navy Bob felt a little sore for a while, but the procedure turned out perfectly. I think he felt fully reassured only when I took his stitches out a week later and he saw for himself that he looked nothing like Frankenstein's monster.[39]

Tragedy at the Tower

A few years before the Beijing 2008 Olympics, the US men's volleyball coach, Hugh McCutcheon, had married Elisabeth Bachman, a star for the US women's volleyball team. By 2008, Elisabeth had retired from active play, but she and her parents joined Hugh in Beijing for the Olympic Games.

The day after the opening ceremony, Elisabeth and her parents, Todd and Barbara, went sightseeing at the Drum Tower near Tiananmen Square, about eight kilometers from the main Olympics site. Without warning, a forty-seven-year-old Chinese man named Tang Yongming attacked the family with a large knife. He killed Todd Bachman on the spot and stabbed Barbara Bachman multiple times. He also stabbed the Bachman family's tour guide. Elisabeth was not injured; she'd been walking a bit ahead of the group when the attack occurred. Chinese security officers responded immediately and prevented anyone else from getting hurt.

Reports vary whether the assailant jumped to his death from a forty-meter-high balcony or was deliberately pushed by security officers. Later reports said the man had recently been divorced and his family had not heard from him for two months.[40]

An emergency medical team stabilized Barbara Bachman at the tower and then rushed her and the tour guide to Peking Union Medical College Hospital, where the trauma team we had arranged to be there executed the trauma plan formulated during the pre-advance visit. They immediately took Barbara to the operating room and saved her life. The tour guide also survived.

I was doing protective medicine duty on the scheduled presidential movement when I heard about the incident through a Secret Service detail. I returned to the RON (remain overnight) hotel and the physician to the president took over the presidential movements.

I, along with Chuck Hartung—a White House nurse who had worked as a critical care nurse in the navy, and who in a few years would become the director of the WHMU—rushed over to Peking Union. We observed the patient, examined the multiple lines and equipment attached to her body, and did our best to decipher the Chinese characters carefully written on various fluid lines. Her medical records, written on paper in Chinese characters, appeared to say that she had received eighty units of packed red blood cells. That seemed like a lot to us, but later we discovered that she had received half units, as compared to the US standard. All in all, she appeared to be getting top-notch care. I returned to President and First Lady Bush, who were personally concerned, and gave them my report.

Once Mrs. Bachman stabilized, the US embassy doctor declared his intention to medivac her to Hong Kong, the next most capable medical facility. But again, I objected. I believed that to transport her to Hong Kong would be a diplomatic gaffe and a source of great embarrassment to China.

When I learned that Mrs. Bachman came from Rochester, Minnesota, I met with the head of the hospital and asked permission for us to medivac her to Rochester, her hometown, which also happened to be the location of the world-famous Mayo Clinic. The suggestion was readily accepted, as I insinuated Peking Union was essentially their Mayo Clinic. I understand that Mrs. Bachman recuperated well physically despite the tragic circumstances.

Once again, we saw that having a plan and following it can save lives. While the life you save may not be the president's, it is equally precious to all family members and friends involved.

The Elevator Incident

Fortunately, not all the memorable moments on presidential trips involve tragedy or high drama.

Hotel elevators always feel tight after a long day of presidential movements. One evening during the 2008 Beijing trip, we returned to the president's hotel, which boasted at least thirty stories. A military aide named Dan Walsh, given the call sign "Scrub," accompanied us. Dan later became the deputy chief of staff at the White House during the Trump administration.

Scrub got in the elevator with his satchel, backed up against the elevator, and unintentionally engaged most of the floor buttons. Unfortunately, that meant that instead of zooming from the ground floor to the designated floor with the presidential suite—usually near or at the top—the elevator proceeded to stop at nearly every floor on the way up.

Scrub had no choice but to take some good-natured ribbing from the president and the First Lady. And if we skipped a floor, everyone in the elevator would yell, "Yippee!"

Always Ready to Provide Care

The physician to the president must remain continually ready to provide superb care to his boss, especially if anything serious happens to him. But the job also means being there for the throngs and multitudes who travel with him . . . while always staying under the radar.

A big part of such care comes in the form of extensive planning for every trip. The White House doctor must make sure that the medical team has the capability to provide on-site care whenever required to whoever in the group may need it, so that together, everyone can continue to care for the president.

That reality prompts me to recall the words of General Eisenhower, who is quoted as saying, "Plans are nothing; planning is everything."

A generation beyond the Reagan assassination attempt, the threats to the health of the president continue. In the twenty-first century, instead of the president's doctor left on the sidewalk, there is a highly trained, prepared, equipped, and experienced team, integrated with the protective detail, ready to promptly respond to trauma, counteract asymmetrical threats, and execute the medical emergency action plan anywhere in the world, ensuring the continuity of the presidency and an enduring constitutional government.

You can't care if you're not there!

THE PURPOSE OF LIFE IS TO
LIVE A LIFE OF PURPOSE

I awoke early on June 12, 2016, a Sunday morning. Almost three years had passed since I left the White House and moved to Orlando, Florida.

The news at daybreak in Orlando horrified me. A man armed with a semi-automatic rifle and pistol apparently had walked past security guards at the Pulse nightclub in the heart of Orlando and went on a murderous rampage. He had driven to Orlando from the Atlantic Coast and had staked out the House of Blues at Disney Springs, but the obvious security apparatus in place there had influenced him to find another target.

So, instead, he headed to the Pulse nightclub, where patrons were celebrating Latin Night. The 320 people inside were getting ready to close it down at last call at about 2:00 a.m. The man let loose his weapons of destruction and over the next three hours left forty-nine individuals dead and fifty-three injured.

In the first few minutes of the attack, many patrons fled. Many who couldn't flee were forced to lie on the ground or barricade themselves in back rooms. The tragedy ranked as the deadliest terrorist attack on US soil since 9/11, as well as (at the time) the most lethal mass shooting in modern US history. Unfortunately, the Las Vegas Strip shooting passed that infamous mark the very next year.

Most of the wounded were rushed a few blocks away to the Level I Trauma Center, Orlando Regional Medical Center, where medical personnel rendered heroic resuscitation efforts and care. Every victim with a heartbeat who entered the trauma center survived and eventually left the hospital. A dozen of the severely injured were taken to AdventHealth Orlando, about four miles to the north, where they also received great care. The nightmare finally ended for some at around 5:17 a.m., when officers working with the Orlando Police Department shot and killed the mass murderer.

As the events unfolded, my mind instantly jumped to the care and travels of the president of the United States, who also serves as the nation's comforter in chief. I knew that President Obama would not want to add to the challenges or overwhelm the law enforcement agencies and medical teams working at the trauma centers and local hospitals. At the same time, however, I felt sure that at the appropriate moment, he would work to give support and comfort to the families of the dead, give hope to the families of the injured, and express his gratitude to law enforcement personnel and to all first responders.

A few days later, Air Force One landed at Orlando International Airport and the president stepped out of the plane and into the Beast. The motorcade moved toward downtown Orlando to the home of the Orlando Magic at the Amway Center. The families of the deceased, some of the injured, and many first responders and law enforcement personnel who had sprung into action that awful day had gathered at the AdventHealth Practice Facility, the Magic's practice basketball court located on the west side of the Amway Center.

With my ties to the president and to Orlando, and because of my personal knowledge of the region's healthcare systems, the physician to the president, Dr. Ronny Jackson (the traveling physician on this trip), reached out and arranged for me to meet with President

Obama after he had completed his duties as comforter in chief. Once the solemn event concluded, the president and I found a quiet place to reconnect. We spent fifteen minutes talking about life. Neither of us asked the other about our travels or work.

"How's your family doing?" both of us asked.

He was very proud of Michelle and his daughters and told me, "They're doing great. One of your patients, Malia, just graduated from high school. And you should be proud, too."

I mentioned the changes in my family and how my wife and four kids had adjusted to a new town and a new school. After our brief time together, the president walked away, then looked back and said, "Thanks for taking care of me and my family."

A TIME OF MAJOR CHANGE

We have reached an era of great generational change, not merely regarding the leaders of our country, but also in corporate America. I believe that the mark of a great leader is to develop those behind him or her so that they can step in and work just as effectively, if not better, than their mentors.

I had the privilege of living among the Greatest Generation (those born between 1901 and 1927) and its leaders for several presidents, up to President George Herbert Walker Bush. And then I was a front-line witness as the leadership and generational mantles were handed over to the baby boomers (those born between 1946 and 1964). Baby boom presidents included Clinton, Bush 43, Obama, and Trump. All were born after World War II and, to one degree or another, reflected the values and culture of their generation. President Biden was born before any of them (in 1942) and so is part of the so-called Silent Generation (made up of those born between 1928 and 1945).

Along with generational changes, we are witnesses to major advances in healthcare, whether the enhancement concerns artificial intelligence, cutting-edge technology, or personalized medicine with tailored treatment targeted to the genetic code of the individual. In view of all such advances, whoever in the future serves as the physician to the president will have to ensure that the doctor-president relationship remains strong and up to date. It must continue to be based on connection and good information and founded on a solid base of trust.

Whoever assumes this key role will quickly discover that the kinship between the president of the United States and the physician to the president has become more relevant than ever.

IT COMES DOWN TO THIS

I've learned that whatever job you have, just do the best you can so long as you're there. You have no idea what the next step will be. A divine leading exists for all of us.

I've also learned that it's better to be lucky than to be good.

For me, it was the privilege of a lifetime to serve in the US Navy for thirty years. And it was the coolest job *ever* to work in both Hawaii and London. Thank you, taxpayers, for financing my overseas adventure of seven years, and then for thirteen years at the White House, where I got to care for the president (and perhaps just as importantly, caring for those who care for the president).

In the end, I think it comes down to this: The purpose of life is to live a life of purpose. Find yours and pursue it with everything in you. You never know where it will lead.

LIST OF PHYSICIANS TO THE PRESIDENT SINCE 1901

President	Physician to the President	Physician to the White House	White House tenure
McKinley & T. Roosevelt	VADM Presley Rixey		1898–1909
Taft	BG Matthew Delaney		1909–1913
Wilson	RADM Cary Grayson		1913–1921
Harding	BG Charles Sawyer		1921–1923
Coolidge	COL James Coupal		1923–1929
Hoover	VADM Joel T. Boone		1922–1933
Franklin D. Roosevelt	VADM Ross McIntyre		1933–1945
Truman	BG Wallace Graham		1945–1953
Eisenhower	MG Howard Snyder		1953–1961
Kennedy	Janet Travell	CAPT George Burkley	
Johnson	VADM George Burkley	CAPT Bill Lukash	
Nixon	MAJ GEN Walter Tkach	CAPT Bill Lukash	
Ford & Carter	RADM Bill Lukash	COL Chester Ward	
Reagan	Daniel Ruge T. Burton Smith BG John Hutton	CAPT Rodney Savage COL John Hutton COL Larry Mohr	
Bush 41	Burt Lee	COL Larry Mohr	
Clinton	RDML Connie Mariano	LT COL Richard Tubb	
Bush 43	BRIG GEN Richard Tubb	CAPT Jeffrey Kuhlman	
Obama	CAPT Jeffrey Kuhlman RDML Ronny Jackson	CDR Ronny Jackson	
Trump	RDML Ronny Jackson CDR Sean Conley		
Biden	COL Kevin O'Connor (retired)		

LIST OF DENTISTS
PROVIDING SERVICE TO THE
PRESIDENT SINCE 1928

Dental Officer (navy, unless otherwise noted)	Presidents
Alfred Chandler, Francis Ulan, William Darnell	Coolidge & Hoover
Arthur Yando	Franklin D. Roosevelt
Bruce Forsyth (USPHS)	Truman
James Fairchild (army)	Eisenhower
John Pepper	Kennedy
James Enoch, Julian Thomas	Johnson
William Chase (civilian)	Nixon
William Maastricht	Ford, Carter
Lawrence Blank, James Judkins	Reagan
Boyd Robinson	Reagan & Bush 41
Roger Doye	Bush 41
Paul Wiley, Scott Haney	Clinton
Austin Maxwell	Clinton & Bush 43
Donald Worm	Bush 43
Evan Applequist	Bush 43
Glenn Munro	Obama

PHYSICIAN TO THE PRESIDENT OFFICIAL TRIP HISTORY

Captain Jeffrey Kuhlman, Medical Corps, Flight Surgeon, US Navy
1/20/2009 to 7/13/2013

Days Available	1,673
Total Trips (days)	420 (697)
Travel Ratio	41.66%
POTUS Trips (days)	413 (683)
Other Trips (days)	7 (14)
CONUS Trips (days)	265 (397)
Overseas Trips (days)	92 (237)
In Town Trips	63

ACKNOWLEDGMENTS

First, thank you to the best collaborative writer in the business, Steve Halliday, and to the entire publishing team at Ballast Books. Thank you!

Anything I have accomplished professionally was built upon the foundation laid out for me by my parents, Henry and Patricia Kuhlman, whether of stability, belonging to a community with a purpose, or the importance of education. I am a poster child and benefactor of a strong Christian education by the Seventh-day Adventist Church. I remember the daily lessons from Mrs. Linebaugh, Mrs. Gorman, and Mrs. Sloan from first to third grade. They skipped me to fifth grade, where Mrs. Halvorson, Mr. Swanson, Mr. Fox, and Mr. Christoph provided me with a stellar education through eighth grade at Arthur W. Spalding Elementary School. For my high school years at Collegedale Academy, I received a great education, with superior teachers and instruction in math, chemistry, biology, history, English, and religion. I also learned that teachers and administrators are human and make mistakes. My twenty-four months of college, with instruction by dedicated professors at Southern Adventist University, prepared me to get into and succeed at medical school at age nineteen. For the third decade of my life, I am grateful to the teachers and clinicians at the Loma Linda University School of Medicine and the Loma Linda University Medical Center who helped me become a competent physician, to listen to every patient, to refuse to become over-enamored with technology, and to give patients something in their time of need.

My first mentor in the navy was Captain Russ Brown, my commanding officer at Naval Hospital Twentynine Palms and again at the US Naval Medical Clinics, United Kingdom. He took a chance on a twenty-six-year-old lieutenant and showed me the navy way of looking out for each other. My first shipmate in the navy was Commander Perry Marshall, who provided me perspective on life and happiness as he lived on his thirty-two-foot Catalina sailboat moored in Pearl Harbor. In London, my fellow naval officers, Matt and Tammy Nathan, were great friends and colleagues. Phil Barham, Danny Carucci, and Jeff Hardin helped open the wonders of London and life; and we remember our friends, Scotty Flink and yeoman warder Peter Hudson.

At HMX-1 the commanding officer sets the pace, runs the show, and flies the president. Thank you, Colonel Ron Berube, for selecting me, and to Colonel Mac Reynolds and Colonel Steve Taylor for their continued confidence and support. Jay Scheiner, Steve Hudson, Brian Hashey, Mark Morris, Chris Frost, Jay Ferguson, Jerome Guansing, Tanya Chalmers, and Marié Thomas—you were an awesome team! The officers and aircrew took wonderful care of me as I did my best to care for them and their families during times of need. Unfortunately, we lost twenty-five marines during my tenure, whether to car accidents, heart attacks, or V-22 mishaps in Arizona and North Carolina. I still think about each one and pray for support and comfort for their families.

I would not have had the opportunity to serve at the White House without the selection, support, and patient guidance of Brigadier General Richard Tubb. Thank you also to the physicians, nurses, physician assistants, healthcare administrators, physical therapists, corpsmen, medics, and support staff of the White House Medical Unit who provided competent medical care to the president, vice president, their families, and the staff who work at the White House. It was an honor and privilege of a lifetime to serve with you from 2000 to 2013.

Thank you, Grace Butler, executive assistant extraordinaire, for your support and advice.

I can't forget to acknowledge the men and women of the Secret Service presidential protective detail and their special agents in charge—Carl Truscott, Eddie Marinzel, Nick Trotta, Don White, Joe Clancy, Mike White, Vic Erevia, and Robert Buster—along with the SAICs of the field offices who I met on the road and in Spare. It was great to work with you all. Speaking of the Spare limo, I need to thank Blake Gottesman, Jared Weinstein, and Reggie Love, the ultimate power forward and friend, and Pete Souza, photographer extraordinaire and my Words with Friends compadre.

The highly competent active-duty directors of the White House Military Office were great to work with. Thank you, Admirals Mike Miller, Mark Fox, and Ray Spicer for your support. The White House mess kept me and the White House fed; thank you to the navy culinary specialists and to Master Chief Tony Powell for your service every day. I learned a lot from the presidential valets. Robert Favela provided valuable assistance in caring for the First Family. During my tenure, I had the privilege to work with fifty military aides to the president and vice president, the cream of the crop of their respective services. Each was a superstar both personally and professionally. The greatest of these was "Navy Bob" Roncska, a tremendous help during the White House days and since. You are high reliability personified.

It takes a global network of medical experts to support the president and his physician. Thank you to Paul Pepe, the world's authority on cardiac arrest and resuscitation; the Eagles Global Alliance; to Don Cook and David Freeman with Shoreland Travax; to Paul Antony, Rear Admiral Connie Mariano, James Gulley of NIH, and Brad Connor and his travel medicine expertise; to Eddie Wasser caring for the Canadian prime ministers; and to highly acclaimed trauma expert Lou Pizano. Thank you, Jack Tsao, for your neurology care with presidents and professional expertise with critical decision-making. I would be remiss if I didn't acknowledge "the Godfather of Medicine" for the national capital region for many decades, Dr. Jim D'Orta; thank you for your helpfulness, guidance, and friendship. I am sure I have forgotten to acknowledge many others. Once I remember, I will regret the omissions and will apologize profusely.

Life is family, faith, and friends. Thank you to my six siblings and their spouses, as well as my eighteen nephews and nieces. My other parents, Michael and Tency Montaperto, and in-laws Vito and Barb, all of you always kept me grounded. Since fifth grade, I have not been able to shake Dennis deLeon, and from the first day of officer indoctrination school, Jim "Aquaman" Marino. Thank you for being lifelong friends. Danny Peach, thank you for a decade of working with me as we help to transform clinical care and save thousands of lives and millions of dollars.

Thank you to my children, Michael, Isabella, Lena, and Henry, who spent their formative years with their father working too many long hours and being absent on trips covering the president and White House travel. Thank you for letting me drag you to yet another Camp David weekend, Easter egg roll, and Christmas party at the White House.

Thank you most of all to my life partner, Sandy Montaperto Kuhlman, who supported me every step of the way and accomplished the impossible job of trying to keep me humble and balanced. Thank you for loving me and caring for me. I would not have accomplished anything professionally or personally without you.

About the Author

Jeffrey Kuhlman served as a navy physician for thirty years, supporting the White House for the last of those sixteen years. He served President Clinton as a Marine One flight surgeon; President Bush as a White House physician, Camp David physician, flight surgeon aboard Air Force One, and director of the White House Medical Unit; and President Obama as the physician to the president. When covering the commander in chief, Dr. Kuhlman was never further than two minutes from the president. In this role, he gleaned personal lessons about the importance of information and relationships built on trust.

As the physician to the president, Dr. Kuhlman coordinated comprehensive healthcare for the president and First Family and oversaw medical care for the vice president (and their family), as well as for senior White House staff and cabinet members. He was also responsible for emergency medical actions and advanced contingency planning, which required collaboration between the White House Medical Unit and the Secret Service protective detail. Dr. Kuhlman provided guidance and advice on all joint service, interagency, and international matters for medical contingency planning and operations. He traveled to more than ninety countries to review their healthcare resources and protocols. His oversight extended to force protection (preventive measures to mitigate hostile actions involving personnel, resources, facilities, and critical information), population health, and workplace health and safety programs for all workers and guests on the White House complex, both at home and abroad.

His mantra: "No politics, no policy, just trusted medical advice."

Dr. Kuhlman attended medical school at the Loma Linda University School of Medicine with residency training at the Loma Linda University Medical Center, the Naval Aerospace Medical Institute, and Johns Hopkins. He completed three clinical board certifications in aerospace, family, and occupational medicine and earned a master of public health degree from Johns Hopkins. He's board certified in medical management, is a certified physician executive by the American Association of Physician Leadership, and is a certified professional in patient safety. His global health expertise includes the certificate of travel health by the International Society of Travel Medicine.

In 2013 Dr. Kuhlman joined the physician executive leadership team at AdventHealth, one of America's largest faith-based health systems, serving as a chief medical officer. Since 2019 he has served as the corporate chief quality and safety officer, extending the healing ministry of Christ.

For the past decade, Dr. Kuhlman has continued to practice primary care medicine, caring for the uninsured, working every month at free and charitable clinics, and spending one to two weeks a year seeing several hundred patients as part of AdventHealth Global Missions. He has traveled multiple times in this capacity to Ethiopia, Peru, the Philippines, and the Dominican Republic.

This is exemplified by his second mantra: "You can't care if you are not there."

ENDNOTES

1   Brian Murphy, "Dennis O'Leary, doctor who updated world after Reagan shooting, dies at 85." *The Washington Post*, February 2, 2022. https://www.washingtonpost.com/obituaries/2023/02/02/dennis-oleary-reagan-shot-dies/.

2   "History of White House Military Office," National Archives and Records Administration, accessed July 16, 2024, https://georgewbush-whitehouse.archives.gov/whmo/history.html.

3   A 2014 study concluded that President Harrison more likely died of septic shock due to "enteric fever," meaning either typhoid or paratyphoid fever. At that time, the water supply for the White House was downstream of public sewage.

4   President Taylor's death was attributed at the time to "cholera morbus," but most experts today think his symptoms point to acute gastroenteritis as the cause of death.

5   Doris Kearns Goodwin, No Ordinary Time (New York: Simon & Schuster, 1994), 491–504.

6   Medically reviewed by Melinda Ratini, "Health Problems of U.S. Presidents," Web MD, January 28, 2023, https://www.webmd.com/a-to-z-guides/ss/slideshow-presidents-health-problems.

7   Christopher Klein, "Did William Howard Taft Really Get Stuck in a Bathtub?" https:www.history.com/news/did-william-howard-taft-really-get-stuck-in-a-bathtub.

8   Ken Johnson et al., "Clinical Evaluation of the Life Support for Trauma and Transport (LSTATTM) Platform." Critical Care 6, no. 5 (July 10, 2002). https://doi.org/10.1186/cc1538.

9   Michael J. Orlich et al., "Vegetarian Dietary Patterns and Mortality in Adventist Health Study 2," *JAMA Intern Med.* 2013; 173 no. 13: 1230-1238, https://jamanetwork.com/journals/jamainternalmedicine/fullarticle/1710093.

10   Atreev Mehrotra and Allan Prochazka, "Improving Value in Health Care—Against the Annual Physical," The New England Journal of Medicine, October 15, 2015, www.nejm.org/doi/full/10.1056/NEJMp1507485.

11   The Cooper Institute. "Legendary 'Father of Aerobics' Dr. Kenneth H. Cooper Turned 90." The Cooper Institute, May 21, 2021. https://www.cooperinstitute.org/blog/legendary-father-of-aerobics-dr-kenneth-h-cooper-turned-90.

12   "Tactical Combat Casualty Care in Special Operations." *Supplement to Military Medicine* 161 (August 1996). An updated edit by Dr. Frank Butler and Dr. John Hagmann in *Supplement to Military Medicine* 165, no. 4 (April 2000).

13   Cybele Mayes-Osterman, "A person in Oregon caught bubonic plague from their cat. Why experts say not to worry," *USA Today*, February 16, 2024, https://www.msn.com/en-us/news/us/a-person-in-oregon-caught-bubonic-plague-from-their-cat-why-experts-say-not-to-worry/ar-BB1ioR02.

14   Tom Ball, "Alexei Navalny was killed 'by punch to the heart,'" *The Times*, February 21, 2024, https://www.thetimes.co.uk/article/1ab5fe9b-d799-4109-bbcb-02c171d96bcd?share-Token=bfc5382dd364b148e67df5bb2b070853.

15   Sarah Beth Hensley and Kevin Shalvey, "Russia to get hit with 'major sanctions' in response to Navalny's death, US says," ABC News, February 20, 2024, https://www.msn.com/en-us/news/world/russia-to-get-hit-with-major-sanctions-in-response-to-navalnys-death-us-says/ar-BB1iAMZO.

16   "Mpox (monkeypox)," World Health Organization, April 18, 2023, https://www.who.int/news-room/fact-sheets/detail/monkeypox.

17   Muriel Lezak et al., *Neuropsychological Assessment*, 5th ed. (New York: Oxford University Press; 2012).

18   NS Wecker et al., "Age effects on executive ability," *Neuropsychology* 14, no. 3 (July 2000), 409–414, https://pubmed.ncbi.nlm.nih.gov/10928744/.

19   Marilyn S. Albert & Mark B. Moss, eds., *Geriatric Neuropsychology* (New York: Guildford Press; 1988), 13–32

20   Vern L. Bengston and K. Warner Schaie, *The Course of Later Life: Research and Reflections* (New York: Springer Publishing Company; 1989), 65-85.

21   B. L. Plassman et al., "Intelligence and education as predictors of cognitive state in late life: a 50-year follow-up," *Neurology* 45, no. 8 (August 1995), https://www.ncbi.nlm.nih.gov/pmc/articles/PMC2683339/#R20.

22   Marja J. Aartsen et al., "Activity in older adults: cause or consequence of cognitive functioning? A longitudinal study on everyday activities and cognitive performance in older adults," The Journals of Gerontology, Series B: Psychological Sciences and Social Sciences 57, no. 2 (March 2022), 153–162, https://pubmed.ncbi.nlm.nih.gov/11867663/.

23   Michael Rönnlund et al., "Stability, growth, and decline in adult life span development of declarative memory: cross-sectional and longitudinal data from a population-based study," Psychology and Aging 20, vol. 1 (March 2005),

24   Timothy Salthouse, "When does age-related cognitive decline begin?" *Neurobiology of Aging* 30, vol. 4 (April 2009), https://www.ncbi.nlm.nih.gov/pmc/articles/PMC2683339/.

25   Knopman, David S, and Ronald C Petersen. 2014. Review of *Mild Cognitive Impairment and Mild Dementia: A Clinical Perspective. Mayo Clinic Proceedings* 89 (10): 1452–59. https://doi.org/10.1016/j.mayocp.2014.06.019.

26   A Mark Clarfield, "The decreasing prevalence of reversible dementias: an updated meta-analysis," Archives of Internal Medicine 163, vol. 18 (October 2003), https://pubmed.ncbi.nlm.nih.gov/14557220/.

27   Davidson, Jonathan R T, et al. 2006. Review of *Mental Illness in U.S. Presidents between 1776 and 1974: A Review of Biographical Sources. The Journal of Nervous and Mental Disease* 194 (1): 47-51. https://doi.org/10.1097/01.nmd.0000195409.17887.f5.

28   Section 7 in the American Psychiatric Association's Principles of Medical Ethics.

29   Vinita Mohta, "Why Some People Think of Pets Like Children and Others Don't," *Psychology Today*, March 27, 2019, https://www.psychologytoday.com/us/blog/head-games/201903/why-some-people-think-pets-children-and-others-dont.

30   Darlene Superville, "Meet Dale Haney, the White House groundskeeper for 50 years," AP, October 24, 2022. https://apnews.com/article/dale-haney-white-house-groundskeeper-35f3c88d2e3e3feedda7db1bfe52f783.

31   Ibid.

32   Ibid.

33   Ibid.

34   Mark Cheathem, "How Martin Van Buren Created the Two-Party System," *The Tennessean*, May 22, 2017. www.tennessean.com/story/opinion/2017/05.22/how-martin-van-buren-created-the-two-party-system/1017612261/. Cheathem is a history professor at Cumberland University and serves as project director for the Papers of Martin Van Buren (VanBurenPapers.org).

35   Tom Shoop, "That Time Abraham Lincoln went to a war zone to escape office-seekers," *Government Executive,* December 27, 2023, www.govexec.com/management12023/time-abraham-lincoln-went-war-zone-escape-office-seekers/3924821.

36   "Lincoln's Visit to Richmond," National Park Service, last updated December 21, 2022, https://www.nps.gov/rich/learn/historyculture/lincvisit.htm.

37   Leah Vredenbregt, "As Biden heads to Israel, looking back at presidents in war zones, from Lincoln to Trump." ABC News, October 17, 2023, https://www.abcnews/Politics/after-bidens-surprise-ukraine-trip-back-presidents-in-war/story?id=97331309.

38   CNN Editorial Research, "2008 Georgia Russia Conflict Fast Facts," CNN, last updated March 13, 2024, https://www.cnn.com/2014/03/13/world/europe/2008-georgia-russia-conflict/index.html.

39   Bob and I are good friends, and we even wrote a book together in 2023 titled *High Reliability Healthcare.*

40   Jessica Mador, "Bachman CEO Killed and Wife Injured in Beijing Attack," MPR News, August 9, 2008, https://www.mprnews.org/story/2008/08/09/bachman-ceo-killed-and-wife-injured-in-beijing-attack.